I0837815

Free Yourself from the Shackles of Fibromyalgia

Free Yourself from the Shackles of Fibromyalgia

Dr. Morgan Sinclair D.C., CFMP
Dr. Casey Sinclair D.C., CFMP

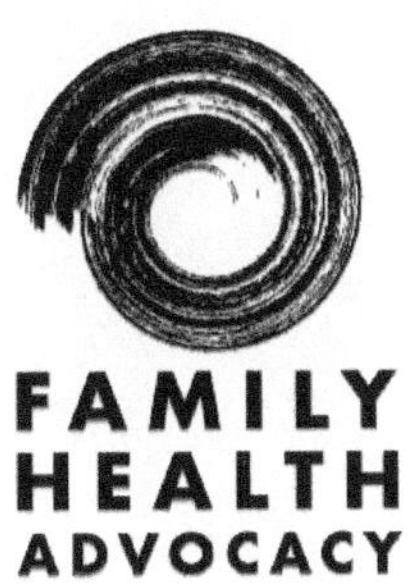

Free Yourself from the Shackles of Fibromyalgia

Family Health Advocacy
Toronto, Ontario
familyhealthadvocacy.com

ISBN: 979-8-62961-391-6

Printed in Canada

Contents

Free Yourself from the Shackles of Fibromyalgia

INTRODUCTION

Fibromyalgia is a chronic pain condition that affects nearly two out of every hundred North Americans. If you broaden the scope to include all people who have chronic pain, the rates skyrocket. Fibromyalgia is so often misdiagnosed, and yet over six percent of the world's population suffers from it. That's over 450 million people, and more than seventy percent of cases are women. The fact that this condition apparently has no known cause or cure has led to more than one million people Googling fibromyalgia every day.

We are Dr. Morgan and Dr. Casey, licensed and practicing Doctors of Chiropractic and certified practitioners of Functional Medicine. We have a wellness-based practice in Toronto, Canada, where we work alongside one another every day. As the son and daughter of a chiropractor, we were raised in a family of holistic healthcare doctors and firmly believe in the body's incredible ability to heal itself, a point this book will continually assert. We are also the founders of Family Health Advocacy, a group led by doctors and health professionals that provides resources and education on global health matters.

Between the two of us, we have been in clinical practice for over twenty years and have served thousands of patients. We witness first-hand the suffering that fibromyalgia causes, as well as the burden it can bring to a whole family. Having dealt with our own chronic pain injuries, we wholeheartedly empathize with our fibromyalgia patients. We have had the privilege of helping countless patients get their lives back using our knowledge of neurology, anatomy, biology, and molecular nutrition. We wrote this book because now we want to help *you*.

One of our greatest passions is helping people be the best versions of themselves—living a truly fulfilling life, doing all the things they love, and enjoying life with their families and loved ones. We inherited this passion from our parents: growing up, we saw our father take such great care of his patients, and our mother has always been mindful of the wellbeing of everyone.

In this book, we endeavor to expose myths and reveal the truth about health and healthcare. Too often, people with fibromyalgia are misled by their healthcare provider and told they cannot be healed. They become shackled by the conditions they are labeled with while feeling condemned to a life of suffering. They're told that the only answer is drugs and surgery.

Everybody has experienced some degree of pain. For those who end up in chronic pain, it often leads to a downward spiral of physical and financial disadvantage along with feelings of social isolation.

There are countless books on fibromyalgia, all with their own take on the condition. Most of these books do not unravel the truth about fibromyalgia, clear up the confusion, or help you understand and address the underlying causes. This book does all of this, while also taking a diverse approach to help you heal. It was written with the belief that you are not helpless or weak, and that there *is* an answer. Your body has an innate intelligence and inherent ability to heal itself if given the opportunity.

Many people suffering from fibromyalgia or related chronic pain are without hope. Many rely on prescription and over the counter drugs, and even sometimes surgery. This book was written to provide those people with hope. You will learn about all areas of healing – from eating the right foods, supplementing for deficiencies, proper exercise, avoiding toxins, and maintaining a well-functioning nervous system – and get proven action steps to lead you to lasting change in order to live a healthy, vibrant life.

The benefits of this book do not end with the last page; it is accompanied by an online course to ensure you have all the right information at your fingertips and can continue to take the right steps to help yourself. Consider this book a launchpad, ready to propel you towards a future of pain-free living. We also invite you to join our online community where we will offer you constant support every step of the way. We believe in you.

Who Is This Book For?

This book is for anyone suffering from or diagnosed with fibromyalgia or similar conditions, such as chronic fatigue syndrome or chronic pain. We wrote it for anyone who is confused by their diagnosis and is looking for real solutions for their symptoms. It's for anyone who is tired of relying on dangerous medications. It's for anyone who wants to understand the true cause of, and cure for, their fibromyalgia.

This book is also for anyone who lives, works, or cares about a sufferer and wants to learn about how they can help. Your support and concern mean so much.

If any of the above describes you, then keep reading. This book is for you!

Who didn't we write this book for? This book was not written for someone who has completely given up.

Chances are, if you picked up this book, that's not you. Congratulations!

The Solution

The solution is never as simple as just one thing. Very few resources address every aspect of fibromyalgia. This book endeavors to do just that.

If you're looking for the solution to health problems including fibromyalgia, you have to address all areas of health including proper mindset, nutrition, supplementation, exercise, toxicity/environment, and the nervous system. This book covers all of that.

Our Promise

Our promise is to support you in making the necessary changes in order to not just restore your health but achieve optimal health. We don't just want you to live – we want you to thrive! We will guide you through with this book, our online course, and our community. We take a relentless approach to most things in life. We are results-driven and solution-focused. This is the approach we take with your health!

About Us

Dr. Casey

I wanted to write this book for those suffering chronically without answers. I know what it's like to be bedridden with pain and immobilized, unable to serve and provide for loved ones. I know what it's like to be in so much pain that you're unable to walk without a cane. Ever laid in bed not knowing if life will ever get better then cried yourself to sleep? I have. I know what it's like when the medical doctor tells you there is no answer other than drugs and surgery. It's incredibly frustrating!

But I also know what it's like to experience all this frustration and emerge from the darkness and despair to see the light! I know what it's like to finally be able to walk normally again, go to work and take care of my patients, play with my children, run, play hockey, and wake surf. I know what it's like to be able to do all the things I never thought would be possible again. Being able to do what I love and love what I do. I know you too can turn your life around, and I want to help you do that.

Dr. Morgan

I started working as a front desk receptionist in my father's chiropractic clinic when I was sixteen years old. I was surprised to learn that so many people live in chronic pain. Aside from bumps and bruises from slips and falls growing up, I didn't really know what chronic pain was. I did, however, understand human emotion. I saw people who had suffered for years before coming into the office, start care, and within weeks or months start to get their lives back. They would tell me about the things they were able to do again. Their ability and love for gardening, biking, downhill skiing was restored. They first came into the office and told me about all the things they thought they would never be able to do again, and now they were doing them with minimal or no pain. I saw lives being transformed. They came from desperation and were restored to health.

The Fibromyalgia Misunderstanding

Fibromyalgia is one of the most misunderstood and misdiagnosed conditions. It is typically characterized by widespread pain in the muscles for a minimum of three months and pain in eleven of eighteen designated tender points. It is associated with joint pain, fatigue, difficulty sleeping, poor concentration, and nervousness. From a medical perspective, there is no known cause or cure. Below is a diagram of where the tender points are located on the body.

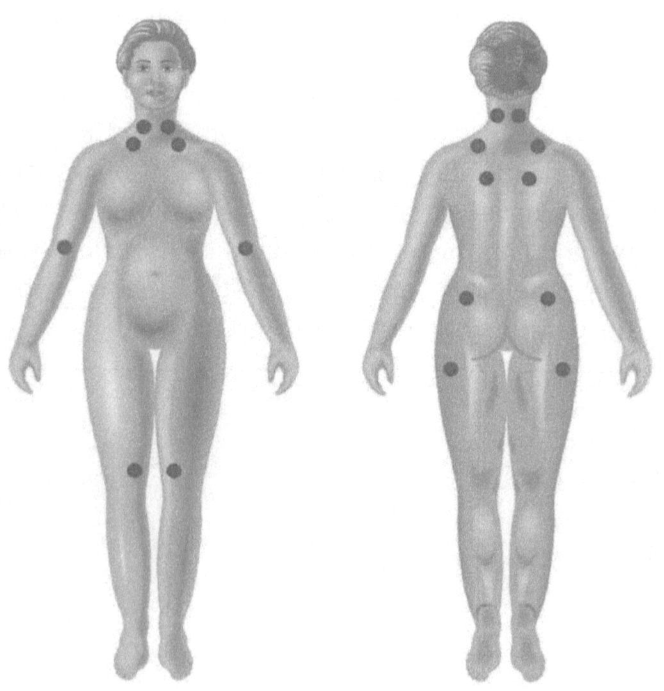

There is no conclusive test to confirm the diagnosis of fibromyalgia. Rather, the diagnosis is based on a process of elimination of other conditions (arthritis, for example). Fibromyalgia is commonly misdiagnosed as muscle and joint pain or myofascial pain syndrome.

The medical community often claims there is no cause for the condition, as well as no cure. However, the FDA has approved three drugs to treat fibromyalgia that we will get into later in this book. If there is no cure, why would there be pharmaceuticals claiming to solve the problem?

Often referred to as a copycat condition, fibromyalgia has many symptoms that make it easy to confuse with different conditions and vice versa. Mix a variety of overlapping symptoms with no definitive diagnostic testing and most doctors are stumped, unable to identify what is causing your aches and pains.

The main symptom of fibromyalgia is widespread pain throughout the body. Fibromyalgia is often referred to as a syndrome, because it is a collection of symptoms that vary among individuals that may or may not include:

Headache	Difficulty Sleeping	Irritable Bowel
Depression	Anxiety	Widespread Body Pains
Painful Menstruation	Arthritis	Restless Legs
Anemia	Stiffness	Fatigue
Overactive Bladder		

…and that's just to name a few.

Acute Pain vs. Chronic Pain vs. Fibro Pain

Acute pain is usually the result of a recent injury or trauma, like spraining your ankle in soccer, having strep throat, or recovering from surgery.

Pain is usually described as chronic if it persists for three to six months, but some doctors use ranges from thirty days to one year for designating pain as chronic. Chronic pain may come and go or be constant, such as low back pain, arthritis in the knees, or pain from an old injury that wasn't treated properly. Typically, there is a specific cause of chronic pain that can be identified (like arthritis) or a herniated disc.

Fibro pain, however, is more of a mystery. It doesn't seem to signal any specific damage. Some people take the diagnosis of fibromyalgia as a curse and become shackled to the diagnosis. The most common myth is that there is no cause for fibromyalgia pain. There is *always* a cause. Many doctors and researchers have examined thousands of possible associations without a definitive answer, but that is because every patient is unique. One theory is that some people have a lower threshold for pain, which would make fibromyalgia exclusively a physical problem. Others believe it is a psychosomatic disorder. What if it's both?

Every individual with fibromyalgia may have a different combination of causes, which is why it is difficult to pinpoint an easy solution. Unlike a disorder with a specific cause and effect, fibromyalgia often requires a complete lifestyle makeover, providing an environment for your body to heal by dramatically decreasing your levels of physical, chemical, and emotional stresses.

Symptoms vs. Condition

Symptoms are red flags your body displays to let you know that there's an underlying problem. Consider them blessings, since it's your body's way of telling you to do something about your health *now*, before it's too late.

Your symptoms are not the problem – they are the manifestation of an underlying problem. Your body develops a problem over time and eventually, the last thing to show up is the symptom.

People typically ignore their symptoms at first, but eventually the body will give you another symptom, and another symptom, until you finally do something about it. That's why some people experience an array of different symptoms—aches and pains all over their body, headaches, digestive problems, fatigue—but it all comes back to the same underlying problem.

If it gets bad enough, some people will try to mask the symptoms with medications, but the drugs are for the symptoms, not the condition. Medication attempts to make you feel better but does not address the underlying cause.

Conditions are the labels medical doctors place on their patients to satisfy the need to have their problem validated, so they have reassurance that it's not all in their head. Many of the labels are just fancy words describing what we already know. The name of the condition doesn't tell you about the underlying problem or cause.

So, when a doctor gives you one of the following diagnoses for your symptoms, what does it really mean?

Fibromyalgia: "Fibro" means fibrous tissue; "my" comes from the word for muscle; and "algia" means pain. So, the word fibromyalgia literally just means a tissue and muscle pain condition. Thanks for telling me what I already know!

Chronic-fatigue syndrome: "chronic" is long-term and ongoing; "fatigue" is tired. So "always tired syndrome." This diagnosis doesn't offer any answers.

Myofascial-pain syndrome: "Myo" is muscle, "fascia" is tissue, and pain…you get it. Muscle-Tissue Pain syndrome! Very enlightening diagnosis!

Sometimes we label a condition by its symptoms. If the diagnosis means nothing, how do we really get to the bottom of your problem?

THE CAUSE. THE CURE.

The Cause

When your body is in a state of chronic dis-ease, caused by stresses of all kinds, disease is inevitable. When you hear the word stress, you automatically associate it with emotions. This is a *huge* misconception. There are many different types of stress. Stress can be physical, chemical, or emotional. The human body is incredibly resilient and allows us to handle stress in all forms to a certain degree. In some cases, stress can even be good for you.

However, in Western culture, we are constantly bombarded with stresses that we were never meant to endure—slumped over our computers and phones all day with poor posture, fighting traffic to and from work, meeting tight deadlines day after day, eating fast food on the run, and so on. All this stress builds up and pushes us beyond our capacity to handle it. When this happens, our body shifts into a state of dis-ease and may present us with signs and symptoms.

Examples of Different Types of Stress

1. **Physical stress** – birthing process, birth trauma, tumbles and falls, sporting injuries, slips, sprains, strains, road traffic accidents, physical labor (repetitive strain), sedentary lifestyle (at a desk/computer or commuting for 40-60 hours/week), sleeping on the couch or an old mattress, sleeping on your stomach or poor sleeping posture.

    Physical stress in the body has a direct physiological effect and often results in inflammation of the joints, muscles, tendons, and nerves. Inflammation is often felt as pain.

    Physical stress causes postural distortion, misalignments of your spine and pelvis, as well as muscle imbalances. If left uncorrected, the problem can complicate and get worse.

2. **Chemical stress** – Medications, preservatives, artificial flavors and colors in our food, antibiotics, hormones, medication and heavy metal residue in our drinking water, personal care products, deodorants, creams, cosmetics,

poor nutrition, shampoo/soap. All of these are toxins that pass through the skin. All increase inflammation and acidity in the body, affect microbiome, and increase pain.

3. **Emotional stress** – Family and work responsibilities, deadlines, financial worries, divorce/breakups, loss of loved ones. We carry all the weight of these stresses on our shoulders and in our nervous system. All of this can increase inflammation and pain.

Nerve Interference

When the human frame is out of alignment, it puts tension and stress on the nervous system, particularly the spinal cord and nerve roots. When the spine is out of alignment it increases dysfunction of the spinal joints, increasing deep inflammation around the nerve roots, dehydrates and damages spinal discs, increasing the rate of spinal degeneration or arthritis. All of this results in even more stress on the spinal cord and nerve roots as well as their corresponding muscles, tissues, organs, and cells. Restricted movement of the spinal joints increases nociception, which in many cases is experienced as pain. When nociceptors (nerve receptors) detect harmful stimuli, pain develops. Restricted joint movement also decreases proprioception which frequently results in even greater loss of coordinated mobility as your awareness of your place in space is diminished.

Poor spinal function leads to poor structure or posture, and poor posture requires increasingly more energy from the brain as it fights to keep your body upright. This can lead to brain fog and symptoms of chronic fatigue and fibromyalgia.

"90 percent of the stimulation and nutrition to the brain is generated by the movement of the spine."
—Nobel Prize winner in Physiology/Medicine,
Dr. Roger Sperry

If the spine is not aligned or functioning optimally, your brain is not receiving proper stimulation. We will show you how this is connected to fibromyalgia symptoms later in this book.

Acute Inflammation vs. Chronic Inflammation

Both stress and nerve interference cause inflammation in the body, and inflammation is linked to both chronic disease and pain. Inflammation in and of itself is not bad. In fact, it is a natural healing response to illness and injury, and in these cases it's usually a short-term condition (days to weeks).

However, when the problem is a dense web of physical, chemical, and emotional stresses, the body is in a *chronic* inflammatory state (months to years). There is a strong connection between this inflammatory state and developing heart disease, cancer, diabetes, arthritis, as well as autoimmune and neurological conditions. A number of studies in recent years are demonstrating the link between chronic inflammation and fibromyalgia.

The Cure

The three types of stress and the inflammation and damage they cause, as well as nervous system interference, all contribute to symptoms of fibromyalgia. If you work to eliminate these causes, your body will be given the space to heal. Before we discuss how to remove the triggers, it's important that you first understand true health.

True Health

True health is not about how you feel or look. The World Health Organization's definition of health is "a state of complete physical, mental and social well-being and not merely the absence of disease or infirmity."

Most people in western culture judge the state of their health based on how they feel and how they look. It's this mentality that causes people to develop health problems and chronic pain. Ask someone who has survived a heart attack, "How did you feel ten minutes before having your heart attack?" They will probably tell you that they felt fine, or even great. And yet they were ten minutes away from having a potentially fatal heart attack. This person might have looked normal and felt fine but clearly not healthy.

Conversely, just because you are experiencing symptoms doesn't necessarily mean you can't heal. Remember we said symptoms can be a blessing: it's your body letting you know there is a problem and giving you the opportunity to find a solution. You just need to learn how to listen.

For example, have you ever hurt your knee? The pain prevents you from running, jumping, walking up and down stairs, crouching, and more. This pain is actually preventing you from doing things that would make the problem worse – it's telling you to take a break in order to heal. Often people will take a muscle relaxant or painkiller to help ease the symptom of the knee pain and allow them to get through the day with more grace and less pain. However, what this is actually doing is fighting the body's natural self-protection mechanism.

Your body is designed to function and heal optimally, as long as you give it the opportunity.

The Body Heals Itself

Your body is a self-healing and self-regulating organism. Much of the time, it doesn't require help from drugs. The master system controlling your body's function and healing is your nervous system. It controls all of the muscles, cells, glands, organs, and tissues. Removing interference to your nervous system and addressing the underlying cause of your problem is the only way to truly heal.

You see, health comes from within us. Remember the time you fell on your knees as a child? You got up and looked down to see your skin was scraped open, smudged with dirt, and highlighted with a drip of blood starting to form. Within seconds your eyes watered up and blurred your vision. You rinsed the area clean with water and covered it up with a Band-Aid. The Band-Aid didn't heal the cut, it simply protected your cut from friction and bacterial invasion.

You didn't have to go to the best doctor in the city to heal. All you needed to do was remove any interference from your body's natural ability to heal, and with time, it would do exactly that.

Your body has the exact same healing ability as it did when you fell and scraped your knee. It has the same ability as it did the day you were born. However, years of physical traumas, emotional stresses, as well as chemical and toxic bombardment has caused interference to your body's innate ability to heal.

For some, trauma, stress, and exposure are layered years deep. For others, the cause will be easier to find. Everyone heals on their own time.

One thing is for certain: if you do what we recommend in this book, you are going to see results. You will find that one day you are doing the things you thought you'd never be able to do again. You'll catch yourself enjoying moments with family and friends that you previously couldn't because of your pain.

If you are willing to put in the work, you will get results. Your health is as important as any other work in your life, because this healing journey is going to take time and energy. Living a life without pain – isn't that worth the effort?

"The doctor of the future will give no medication but will interest his patients in the care of the human frame, diet and in the cause and prevention of disease."
—Thomas A. Edison

You must address all areas of your health in order for your body to fully heal. This includes:

- Mindset
- Nutrition
- Exercise
- Environment / Toxicity
- Nervous System

It's easy to focus on only one thing and neglect the rest, but the problem needs to be approached holistically, from all angles. Fibromyalgia can be due to a deficiency in any or all aspects of your health, so it's important to address them all, which we will attempt to cover in this book.

The Problem

Our Healthcare System Is Really a Sick Care System

North America has incredible resources, cutting-edge technology, and well-trained doctors to handle crisis care situations. We have one of the best emergency care systems in the world. All of this is amazing, and we should be grateful. The problem? A very small percentage of all the drugs consumed and surgeries performed are part of that emergency critical care system. Most treatments referred to as "lifestyle" drugs and surgeries are used for patients with chronic conditions and diseases that are a result of many poor health choices. These treatments are essentially band-aid "solutions" to mask symptoms and do nothing to solve the underlying problem. The folly of our sick care system is its refusal to acknowledge that we can't medicate our way out of conditions that we've "life-styled" our way into (knowingly or unknowingly). The medical system has limited options. It's literally a two-trick pony. 1) Drugs, 2) Surgery. That's it. Neither of these options acknowledges or honors your body's innate ability to heal. People are tired of this approach and are searching for an answer. This book opens the door to unlimited health opportunities.

Betty's Story

I'm 60 years old, and at one point was very ill and experiencing poor organ function. I've had to deal with car accidents and other injuries over the years.

I started to feel better very quickly following the advice from Dr. Morgan and Dr. Casey.
I am now able to do things quite simply that were at one time hard. I'm able to do things that I at one time took for granted, such as walking, driving a car, getting in and out of the bathtub, but most importantly, getting down on the floor to play with my grandchildren. My body now feels in alignment and powerful, and I'm feeling young again!
I recommend this program to anyone as it has been such a blessing to my life.

HEALTHY MIND

The most important aspect of your health begins with your mindset. Fibromyalgia symptoms in both women and men can overlap with psychosomatic disorders, and the symptoms usually start with pain, headaches, nausea, or sleep disturbances, and can evolve into depression and anxiety. We are not saying that fibromyalgia is a mental problem – we are saying that it can *lead* to one. Fibromyalgia has commonly been categorized as a chronic central nervous system disorder, but research suggests a strong correlation between fibromyalgia and mental health.

Stress Biology & Fibromyalgia

One of the underlying causes of fibromyalgia is chronic stress. A fundamental understanding of the effects stress has on your body will help you take the necessary steps to be proactive in reducing life's stressors.

When researchers placed stem cells in the presence of stress hormones, their immunity and growth immediately declined, and the cells died. The same thing happens in our bodies. But once stress is removed, normal growth and healthy immunity resumes.

Many of us live in a state of chronic stress, and this is especially true of fibromyalgia patients who experience high physical, emotional and/or chemical stress.

When in this state of stress, vital energy is redirected in the body to help adapt to the stressful circumstance. Cells are deprived of energy as the blood is redirected to the musculoskeletal system. Blood is also squeezed out of our forebrains, reducing rational thinking, and concentrated in our hind brains for reflex behavior as we defend for ourselves. This is our fight or flight instinct. When we are in this survival mode, energy to our immune system is reduced in order to prioritize the external stressor, and the internal stress, such as fighting an infection, is no longer a priority.

As a result, cellular growth and immunity is compromised while in a state of stress, setting the stage for sickness and disease. Historically, stress has been transient and episodic, but as mentioned, today we live in a society with constant chronic stress. This is reflected in the fact that pharmaceutical drug sales increased by twenty percent immediately after 9/11. When the nervous system perceives an environmental threat, it starts the process of secreting fear hormones throughout our body so that we start to feel the way we think and think the way we feel. Cells only respond to the nervous system's perception of our environment. If our perception of the environment is exaggerated or distorted, then the effects of stress begin to proportionately compound.

While it is not possible to avoid stress entirely, it's important to change your perception of how you see your stress in life. As they say: if you can't change your environment, you can change your attitude.

Mindset

Many people who see doctors about chronic pain have been told that it's all in their head. We do not agree. The pain is very real.

What *is* in your head is the powerful ability to re-wire how your brain perceives pain, which can be an output from the brain rather than an input from the body. For someone experiencing chronic pain, the brain can perceive light touch as being painful, but you can learn to control your brain's perception.

The key to removing one of the biggest and most common forms of interference is understanding how the mind, not just the body, is responsible for your experience of chronic pain. Thoughts and events from the past and present have an impact on our physical health. There are widespread neurological implications caused by emotions like anger, anxiety, fear, self-doubt, the sense of failure, and more. Outside therapies like massage therapy or supplements, although helpful, are somewhat limiting. When you don't remove negative conscious and subconscious thought patterns your emotions will continue to govern your body. Instead, you need to learn how to manage your emotions, and therefore control your healing.

Pain is an experience. Physical pain from an external stimulus will trigger a message to be sent from tissues, through neurons called nociceptors, to the brain in order to alert to a potentially dangerous situation. This message arrives at the brain and its level of "danger" is determined by your brain's conditioned learned response from life's experience. Your brain and nervous system form memories of painful experiences. This helps us avoid behavior that once resulted in pain, like touching a hot stove.

We also create painful memories that we imagine and perceive from the pain of others. If you have ever been diagnosed with a pinched nerve you have already created a "pinched nerve" memory in your brain. Your brain has a context of what a pinched nerve means based on any experience related to the diagnosis. Brain cells in the "pinched nerve" memory bank will also belong to anything else you associated the pinched nerve diagnosis with—neck pain, numbness, tingling, weakness, sciatica, and so on. This means if you are told you have a pinched nerve, you activate the brain cells associated with a pinched nerve and experience its symptoms, even if you don't really have a pinched nerve. This is one of the dangers of a misdiagnosis. This information – often inaccurate – that we have gathered about how we imagine our body to work has contributed to our brain's evaluation of how much danger we are in, and therefore affects perception and experience of an external pain stimulus.

Now, we will work through some relevant and applicable mindset concepts that you can start to apply today in order to change your perception of your pain. Each concept is accompanied by paradigm-shifting exercises.

We are going to cover some time-tested practices of emotional healing:

- Gratitude
- Affirmations
- Acknowledging your achievements

The more energy and time you put into these exercises, the more you will get out of them. You will soon see how your mind can't tell the difference between reality and what you tell it. This chapter is one that you may need to re-read a few times and will revisit time and again.

Some patients are more prepared than others to challenge their state of mind during their healing process. We provide guidance in the form of literature, counseling, and advanced workshops on developing a healthy mindset. It's not uncommon to see patients with very similar symptoms in our practice. However, the patients who dedicate the time and energy to their mental health and creating a positive mindset tend to get better results with their care. The positive mindset they cultivate drastically decreases their healing time and ability to return to normal activities of daily living, pain-free.

Gratitude

The feeling of gratitude can be the foundation of your healing. Gratitude truly allows you to create your reality. Over the past ten years in our private practice, we have witnessed the profound connection between gratitude and healing in our patients. In our opinion, it is one of the major principles of health.

Gratitude is a tool that can be an extremely powerful force in healing both your mind and body. When patients are in a state of frustration, despair, anger, or resentment about their condition, they often slip into a victim mentality with little faith in their ability to self-heal.

Gratitude, on the other hand, has the effect of lightening the load. The body has an innate intelligence and an incredible healing ability. Allopathic treatments and remedies have their place, but if you are relying solely on them, you will be unable to fully experience your body's innate ability to heal. These treatments simply support your *own* natural healing processes.

The principle of this gratitude practice is that you must trust that you will heal. It's easy to imagine the worst-case scenario, but instead, practice imagining the *best-case* scenario. This simple mental shift will change everything. Every day take time to visualize yourself doing what you love and loving what you do in a state of gratitude because you are healthy.

Our family introduced us to gratitude journals at a young age. Not only has it helped us keep a strong sense of gratitude through the challenges of life, but we have introduced the concept to our patients with great success. This practice helps people get their heads into a space of love and appreciation for their lives as they are. Remember, you can't always change your circumstance, but you can change your attitude.

For someone going through a dark season in their life or struggling with chronic pain, doing the following gratitude journal exercise may feel difficult, time-consuming, and useless at first. We encourage you to stay committed. After planting a flower seed, with daily sunlight and watering it still takes weeks to see the plant emerge from the soil. Be patient. Everything takes time, and so does healing.

You can find a gratitude journal to practice at https://familyhealthadvocacy.com

Step 1: Find a blank notebook or journal and a pen. We recommend using a fresh book so the only thing inside is gratitude.

Step 2: Dedicate special gratitude journal time right before bed. Place the journal next to your bed on your nightstand.

Step 3: When night falls, reflect on your day. Write three things that happened throughout your day that you are grateful for. Relish life's simple pleasures like the delicious healthy breakfast you had, or the five minutes spent in the yard breathing the fresh crisp air and feeling the heat of the sun on your back. Reflect and be grateful for even more memorable moments, like spending time with a friend, a family get-together over the holiday, or the celebration of life's successes.

Step 4: This is the final and most important step—repeat these steps every day. If you happen to miss a day, the next day write six things you are grateful for.

Cherry on top: Over time, you will have a journal filled with reasons to be thankful for what you have and enjoy. On days you are needing a reminder or inspiration, open the journal and spend time reminding yourself of what you are grateful for, and your life's pleasures.

"The more you are grateful for what you have, the more you will have to be grateful for."

—Zig Ziglar

Affirmations

Affirmations are positive sentences or declarations used to train both your conscious and subconscious mind. By regularly repeating these affirmations, you condition your subconscious mind in order to influence the desired behavior, habit, or action. Affirmations are designed to keep you positive, motivated, inspired, and focused on your goal.

Affirmations affect your brain on a cellular level by disrupting your negative thoughts and old ways of thinking. You become rewired with your new affirming beliefs. The scientific concept behind this is called neuroplasticity.

"Your thoughts have a direct connection to your health."
—Dr. Joe Dispenza,
Physics, The Brain, and your Health.

Simply put, neuroplasticity is the brain's ability to form new neural pathways, firing and wiring in new patterns, sequences and combinations resulting in new thoughts.

It takes time to create your own affirmations that are unique to you. It's worth it. An affirmation you create that is specific to your own life will be much more powerful than using one you find.

How to do Affirmations

1. Make note of the negative beliefs you have about yourself. Example: "I don't exercise because I'm too busy and tired."
2. Reframe those negative beliefs and write them as a positive statement about yourself. Example: "I make time to exercise every day because it provides me with more energy to get more things accomplished."
3. Your affirmation is personal to you! Start with the word "I," and follow with an action word: I make, I do, I am.
4. State your affirmation in the present tense. State it as if it's already a reality.
5. Make it about what you want, not what you don't want.
6. Brevity is brilliance and simplicity reigns supreme here. Keep your affirmations short, succinct, and to the point.
7. Include one dynamic emotion or feeling word.
8. Make your affirmations for yourself.

Here are some more examples of affirmations you can be inspired by to help you with reframing your perception of pain:

- I am on a healing journey and I feel great.
- I make time every day to prioritize my wellness.
- I do exercises with my body and my mind which have rewired my brain and changed my perception of pain.
- I deserve this feeling of energy and great health.

Take time every day to repeat your affirmations. Say them aloud with high energy and enthusiasm. Stand up when you do your affirmations. If you have a hard time focusing, try closing your eyes when you repeat them. The best time to repeat your affirmations are early morning and throughout the day when you need a reminder of your focus. Again, be persistent and patient as research shows that a minimum of thirty days of affirmations are required before you begin to see a measurable change in the reprogramming of your subconscious mind.

Acknowledge Your Achievements

Take time at the end of each day to reflect and recognize your achievements. This will keep you motivated in achieving your long-term goals. Give yourself the opportunity to enjoy the sense of success, and the joy and satisfaction that comes from that. Acknowledge not just your ability to reach certain goals, but your dedication and commitment throughout the process of reaching those goals! All of this will contribute to your personal growth and cultivate positive emotions that are crucial for healing.

Two ways to acknowledge your achievements:

1. Achievement journal – Record every win, big or small, in your journal. As your accomplishments pile up, review your journal and reflect on all of your victories. Wins and accomplishments can be as simple as getting out of your pajamas one day, or as big as going for a two-hour hike.

2. Rewards – Each time you achieve a goal, reward yourself. Buy yourself a new outfit or piece of jewelry or enjoy a night out. Allow these rewards to remind you of your success every day.

Lucas's story

I struggled with fibromyalgia for over 20 years. It all started when I had a stressful year at work. I was pulling off ten-hour days with no breaks, five days a week at a minimum. Suddenly, after eight months of working on a project at work, I came down with a series of flu-like symptoms and infections. I struggled with widespread muscle aches, fatigue, and weakness in my arms and legs. I pushed through with this seemingly chronic flu and continued to work for about two months. The symptoms never went away; they simply got a little better or worse. One morning I was pouring milk into my tea and I dropped the carton. That was the tipping point. I drove to work that day and applied for a leave of absence. Simple activities of daily life were now a challenge. I was failing miserably as a caregiver and friend to my two children and spouse.

I started bouncing from doctor to doctor receiving a battery of tests. I was given many referrals, but never any answers. My family doctor and I felt at a loss. She eventually diagnosed me with fibromyalgia.

Every chore around the house and outing with my kids became a huge task. It took five times as long to recover than it would to participate in a family activity. I felt like I had become a burden. I made a last-ditch attempt to have hope and health in my life by attending a health seminar with my neighbor. It was a half-day seminar that completely turned my life around. I met other people who had struggled just like I was, but these people had gotten their lives back. I left there with an appointment to have special testing done. I also left inspired and finally felt hope again. After my initial appointment with Dr. Morgan and Dr. Casey, they scheduled me for detailed sessions to discuss my results with a focus on removing the underlying causes of my symptoms. Everything became clearer. Once some of my underlying issues were dealt with over the following three months, I began to feel energized and strong. I felt like I finally had control of my body and I was given a second chance at life. Ten months after I started their program, I completed the annual five kilometre walk held in my town. The best part about this accomplishment is that I completed the walk alongside my children.

I finally wake up in the morning excited for the day. The years of struggling with my health are in the past.

A HEALTHY BODY

Nutrition is an essential component of healing. When we eat a balanced diet and prioritize foods rich in vitamins and minerals, our bodies run like properly functioning machines. Making poor food choices is like putting water in a gas tank: your body will only run for so long.

In this chapter you will find information on some foundational nutritional concepts, and clear guidance on what steps to take to make a change. *Bon appétit*!

Leptin Resistance and Fibromyalgia

A key factor in many chronic pain syndromes is an imbalance of leptin, a hormone that tells your brain to burn fat and regulates your appetite. When leptin levels rise, the brain gets a signal to tell you you're full, so you stop eating, and you burn fat. When your leptin levels are chronically spiked, you become resistant to leptin. This means the brain can't hear the message anymore and becomes less responsive to the hormone. When the brain doesn't sense leptin, it doesn't get the signal that you are full. Therefore, the brain thinks you're starving, and you end up eating more while the body stores energy from digested food. This makes burning or oxidizing fat difficult.

Here's an analogy: if you have just moved into a home on a busy street, you will initially be surprised and disturbed by all of the loud noises. Every time a car horn honks, or a bus goes by, you will notice and be irritated. However, over time, the noises will become so familiar that they will be background noise. People visiting you will notice, but you won't even be able to hear what they're talking about. Your body will have developed a resistance in order to protect yourself from the constant irritation.

The same thing happens with leptin. When there is an overload of leptin in the bloodstream constantly telling the brain "Burn fat! Burn fat!" the brain eventually ignores those signals and you gain weight. Your body is still producing leptin, but your brain is not listening. As a result of your brain thinking that you are starving, the body can go into a low-energy state and experience fatigue, brain fog, and weakness.

Research shows that refined sugar is a leading cause of leptin resistance. Focus on avoiding refined sugar from junk foods, sweetened drinks, and condiments. Avoid eating refined carbohydrates such as white rice and bread, and instead eat whole grains and complex carbohydrates. Eat fruits that are low in fructose like lemons, limes, grapefruit, kiwis, and berries. Appropriate exercise also has a huge impact on leptin.

When you repair your leptin receptors and are no longer in a resistance state, you will decrease cravings and increase energy.

Mark's Story

I'm 28 years old and have been working in sales for the last five years. I had been in two car accidents, which I believe contributed to my widespread body pain. Some days the pain was so brutal that I couldn't walk. I was at the point where I thought I would never live a normal life again. I was very skeptical about following the doctors' protocol but decided it was my last chance. I'm so glad I took it!

All of my pain is gone. I have regained so much mobility and flexibility and I can now walk with ease. I am now able to go to the gym and work out. My overall quality of life has improved so much. I found the doctors to be really helpful and they took the time to explain everything. I now have a great understanding of how the body is designed to work!

I recommend this program to anyone looking to increase their quality of life and just getting out there and doing all the things they love. It's amazing the changes that can occur when taking care of your body and maintaining proper nutrition.

Antioxidants, Free Radicals, and Oxidative Stress

We hear so much about the importance of antioxidants to our health. Most of us know enough about free radicals to know that they are bad, and some of us are also familiar with oxidative stress. Let's get into detail to really understand these concepts and what they do.

Every day, our bodies are blasted with different types of stress. People grab meals on-the-go in the form of processed or fast foods. We are exposed to environmental toxins in the air both inside and outside of our homes. People are overworked and overstressed, sitting at their desks and computers for forty to sixty hours a week, trying to meet the next deadline. As a result of all this work, it's hard to find time to get any exercise. All these stressors lead to the buildup of oxygen-containing toxic waste in the body. These are known as free radicals.

A free radical is an unstable atom. Your body is made up of trillions of cells and your overall health depends on the health of those cells. The cells are healthy when made up of stable atoms.

A stable atom has two paired electrons on its outer shell. An unstable electron only has a single unpaired electron. This free radical empty space left by the missing electron will be taken up by the toxic waste generated by all the stressors in your daily life. To avoid this, the single electron atom starts looking around at other stable atoms in healthy cells to steal an electron to fill its empty void.

The stealing of electrons from other stable atoms leads to cell breakdown. As the number of free radicals increases, the cells break down even further. This is called oxidative stress. This process is connected to every aspect of your health. Oxidative stress in your body is very similar to that of a rotting apple. Picture an apple that has been sliced in half and left on the counter. As it continues to be exposed to the oxygen in the room, the inside of the apple begins to turn brown and decompose.

Oxidative stress leads to conditions like cardiovascular disease, cancer, accelerated aging, a weakened immune system, and a compromised nervous system. We cannot completely avoid free radicals and oxidative stress, but we can offset their impact on our health by ensuring a healthy daily consumption of antioxidants. The best way to ensure ample antioxidant consumption is through proper nutrition and supplementation.

What are Mitochondria and Why are they so Important?

The body is made up of trillions of cells and relies on energy so each cell can perform its proper function. This energy is created in the mitochondria of the cells.

The mitochondria convert food into a chemical energy known as ATP (Adenosine Triphosphate). The mitochondria then release this energy into the cell where it can be used.

Think of a windmill converting wind into energy that supplies energy to your town. Dysfunction of the mitochondria can lead to pain, fatigue, and many other fibromyalgia symptoms. Many studies suggest that in addition to oxidative stress and inflammation, mitochondrial dysfunction plays a significant role in fibromyalgia symptoms. Mitochondria are easily affected and damaged by poor nutritional choices, exposure to toxins, trauma, pharmaceutical drugs, and stress. Lifestyle and proper supplementation help restore proper mitochondrial function.

Now that you have a better understanding of leptin, antioxidants, free radicals, oxidative stress, and mitochondria, let's discuss the glycemic index and the role of insulin.

Glycemic Index and Insulin

When you eat, your body breaks down carbohydrates and converts them to a type of sugar called glucose. Glucose is the main source of energy for our cells. The time it takes for the body to convert food into glucose and release it into the bloodstream varies depending on the food source. The bloodstream is the delivery system for the glucose to be delivered to where it's needed. Insulin, which is released by the pancreas, is the chauffeur for glucose. It guides the glucose from the bloodstream and into the cells for use or storage.

Some foods cause the blood glucose level to rise rapidly, while others are converted and delivered into the bloodstream more gradually. The glycemic index is a measurement of how quickly – and by how much – a food raises blood glucose levels. High glycemic index food raises blood sugar rapidly. Low glycemic index foods raise blood sugar levels more slowly, and to lower levels. Low glycemic index food gives the body time to process the glucose more effectively.

Think of feeding a child Lucky Charms cereal for breakfast. They'll have an instant sugar high and then be hungry very soon after eating. If you feed them scrambled eggs instead, they will be full for longer and won't have the sugar spike and crash.

When blood sugar rises quickly, the pancreas kicks into gear and releases insulin to get rid of excess glucose in the bloodstream and guide it into storage inside of cells. If you regularly eat high glycemic index foods and cause the blood sugar levels to spike often, you consistently trigger your pancreas to produce insulin to bail you out of blood sugar poisoning. Eventually, cells get tired of insulin knocking at their doors and do not open. When this happens, cells have become resistant to insulin.

Insulin resistance leads to many more problems:

1. Chronic high blood glucose, or prediabetes
2. Fatigue and a craving for carbohydrates as a result of cells not receiving glucose, which is referred to as hypoglycemia
3. The pancreas produces more insulin and delivers it to the bloodstream resulting in a chronically high insulin state, which in turn results in energy going into fat storage rather than being used for energy at a cellular level
4. Insulin resistance may also be a risk factor for memory impairment with people who suffer from fibromyalgia

If you have musculoskeletal pain or headaches in addition to blood sugar issues, you can easily see how the combination of symptoms can mimic or be misdiagnosed as fibromyalgia. Insulin resistance can, however, be corrected with proper sleep, healing nutrition, and exercise.

Denise's Story

I am a 30-year-old preschool teacher. I used to be in so much pain that life was awful and unbearable. I was sick a lot and would frequently miss work, so this was affecting me financially. I was often irritable. I was also getting headaches which I felt were ruining my life. I would miss a lot of birthdays and weddings with friends and family because I was in so much pain. I had gone to so many doctors but there were no answers. I was always told to take different medications which never worked. I was diagnosed with diabetes and was on medication, but nothing changed.

I was truly skeptical of this program, but it was my only option left. For the past three years, I am proud to say that I haven't missed a single day of work! I am off my medication. I rarely get headaches and am feeling so much better overall. I truly feel I am in safe hands with Drs. Morgan and Casey. Their care and protocol are the only thing that has ever worked for me.

NUTRITION

Sugar

Sugar is responsible for the obesity epidemic in North America. Sugar consumption leads to lower immunity and has been linked to diseases ranging from metabolic syndromes, chronic fatigue, diabetes, headaches, cardiovascular disease, ADHD, cancer, depression, and of course inflammation and chronic pain syndromes.

Sugars and simple carbohydrates are easy go-to foods when on the run or too tired to prepare a meal. A pack of candy may provide you with a quick bump of energy, but it will cost you more energy in the long run. High glycemic index foods will raise your blood sugar fast and then drop it quickly, resulting in reactive hypoglycemia. Sugar has no nutritional value, and it even depletes nutrient stores because the body needs to use energy to heal from the havoc sugar creates.

Are you an addict? Just like cocaine, people can have a strong addiction to sugar. Most people don't even know it. Sugar, like many other substances or habits, stimulates the feel-good hormone dopamine. Some researchers believe people addicted to sugar should be treated in the same way as people addicted to drugs.

Sugar metabolically shifts your body from a fat-burning machine to a sugar-burning, energy-storing state. It swings your body into starvation mode. Even though you have plenty of energy stored, your cravings for more sugar remain.

Remember when we discussed leptin resistance? Sugary foods raise insulin and leptin levels significantly, eventually leading to insulin and leptin resistance. Eliminating sugars allows for your body to heal from the resistance and return to homeostasis, or a balanced state.

A nutrition plan eliminating sugars for a period of time is necessary to allow for leptin and insulin levels to be regulated and receptors to heal. Eventually, you will be able to re-introduce healthier natural sugars in moderation. When leptin and insulin levels are restored, your body will shift back to a fat-burning and energy-using machine and your appetite will regulate. This means you will have more energy, and the fatigue associated with your fibromyalgia will decrease, your muscles will be stronger, and your cravings will be minimized.

Sugar is also fuel for the overgrowth of yeast. Many types of bacteria and yeast live in our bodies that are essential to the immune system. Candida Albicans is a fungus that normally lives on our skin and in the gastrointestinal tract and it aids with nutrient absorption and digestion without causing any problems. But high sugar intake is like pouring gasoline on a controlled fire resulting in Candida overgrowth and yeast infections.

Recent or frequent antibiotic use can also contribute to an infection because it creates an imbalance of the natural bacteria and yeast. Overgrowth of yeast in the body can be a cause of widespread inflammation. Yeast or Candida overgrowth can be difficult to diagnose as it presents in various ways. Many of the symptoms are similar to those of fibromyalgia, including lowered immunity, presenting as frequent common colds or sinusitis, fatigue, digestive symptoms, hormonal imbalances, vaginal yeast infections in women, changes in mood and difficulty concentrating referred to as brain fog or "fibro-fog."

Testing for overgrowth of yeast can be done with a blood test or fecal sample. Treatment includes eliminating sugars and carbohydrates in addition to taking a quality probiotic supplement. Check out our top recommended probiotics at:

familyhealthadvocacy.com

It's easy to point out sources of sugar in the convenience store like candy, soda, chocolate bars, and sugar-coated cereals, but there are hidden sources of sugar in things we consume regularly. Crackers, bread, energy bars, flavored yogurt, pizza, and fruit drinks are just a few foods with hidden sources of sugars. Even foods promoted as "healthy" or "natural" can be layered with sugars.

According to the U.S. Department of Agriculture, the average annual consumption of sugar per person in 2015 was 94 grams per day, which adds up to 76 pounds per year. That is more than a five-pound bag of sugar each month. This is crazy!

It's difficult for consumers to truly understand the sugar content in food sources because of confusing labeling guidelines. The Nutrition Facts label does not list "added sugars" due to the manufacturer's difficulty in determining the amount of added sugars in a food or drink. During processing, some sugars are converted to other ingredients.

More important than the Nutrition Facts is the Ingredient List. You will find any and all added sugars here. Ingredients are listed in the order of weight, from most to least. Manufacturers can also easily disguise the layers of sugar in the product by listing them as different names. There are at least fifty-seven different names for sugar that they can use.

Common sugars or aliases found in ingredient lists include:

Sucrose	Corn sweetener
Evaporated cane juice	Agave nectar
Barley malt	Maltodextrin
Fructose	Fruit juice
Honey	Concentrates-glucose
Dextrose	Lactose
Raw sugar	Cane crystals
Maple syrup	Crystalline fructose
Invert sugar	Malt syrup
Maltose	Cane sugar
White sugar	Brown sugar
Rice syrup	Isomalt
Sugar syrup	Caramel
Rice malt	

So, if the manufacturer lists the sugars as separate ingredients, the overall quantity of sugar is divided and will be spread throughout the ingredient list in order to appear less offensive.

This doesn't mean all so-called "sugar-free" products are safe, though. Read the label! Often aspartame is added to sugar-free products, which is a neurotoxin that has a major negative impact on your health. Stay away from sugar and even further away from Aspartame.

Grains

Grains are rarely found as whole grains anymore: in our supermarkets, they usually come highly processed for convenient consumption which results in the loss of their nutritional value. In North America, consumption of processed grains is higher than ever before. They are cheaper to manufacture and have a longer shelf life. Compare the five-day shelf life of an organic whole grain loaf of bread, free of preservatives, to that of pre-sliced white Wonder Bread at thirteen or more days of shelf life. It's easy to see how someone who doesn't understand the negative health impact of consuming processed refined grains can be swayed by the long shelf life and low price point.

Consumers love refined grains because they are easy to prepare and have become a staple with many meals. Refined grains typically have a higher glycemic index and turn to sugars in your digestive tract, which contributes to the sugar cascade and results in inflammation.

There are health benefits to grains if they are whole grains. Whole grains maintain a higher nutrient and fiber value and provide a steady energy source as a result of their low glycemic index value. Sprouted and fermented grains are good whole grain options. However, if your goal is to get more fiber in your diet, a better source of complex carbohydrates is vegetables. Vegetables are also loaded with nutrients. Gluten is a protein present in most grain and wheat products and it can be difficult to digest, especially for those with food sensitivities. Gluten can cause inflammation in the body and is found in pasta, bread, crackers, white rice, cereals, and other grain products. The repetitive onset of inflammation contributes to many chronic diseases and conditions including fibromyalgia.

Symptoms of gluten sensitivity can be different for each individual and can present themselves in varying degrees. Many of these symptoms are similar to those of fibromyalgia, including brain fog, weight loss resistance, migraines, headaches, fatigue, irritability, mood changes, depression, lack of muscle control, chronic muscle pain, digestive problems like bloating, and widespread inflammation leading to increased pain.

In our clinical experience, we have observed that many patients have had a noticeable decrease in pain when they eliminate gluten from their diet. A study in *Rheumatology International* found that patients with fibromyalgia achieve significant improvement by eating a gluten-free diet. The research suggests that a "non-celiac gluten sensitivity may be an underlying treatable cause of fibromyalgia syndrome."

If you experience the symptoms listed above, we recommend a six-week gluten-free nutrition plan. You may feel noticeably different after a few days, or you may not feel any different after a few weeks, but either way, we suggest following through the full six weeks to get an accurate test for sensitivities. If at the end of six weeks you do not notice any changes in your health and well-being, try eating a product with gluten and make note of any changes in your mood, digestion, and energy levels. If your symptoms flare up, then you most likely have a gluten sensitivity or intolerance.

Countless studies and research support the fact that your nutrition affects your overall health. Consuming sugar, processed grains, and other inflammatory foods wreaks havoc on your body. Gluten actually damages the lining of the digestive system, leading to a lack of nutrients being absorbed, such as vitamin B12 and all fat-soluble vitamins, which are often deficient in fibromyalgia sufferers.

Symptoms of gluten sensitivity:

- Digestive problems (bloating, constipation, diarrhea)
- Fatigue
- Sleep disturbances
- Brain fog ("fibro-fog")
- Weight gain
- Widespread pain
- Headaches/migraine

- Yeast infections
- Acid reflux/GERD

All of the gluten sensitivity symptoms are very similar to those of fibromyalgia. Is it becoming more clear how important nutrition is to your health and well-being? Do you feel empowered, knowing that your diet is within your control?

Helma's Story

Over 15 years ago, I suffered from back pain. It was so painful that I was unable to go to the gym, something I loved doing. I was constantly tired and always reaching for food, hoping it would increase my energy. I essentially became a sugar addict. I was sedentary, tired, making bad food choices, and spiraling into poor health. The pain never went away and was getting worse. I was frustrated and tired of it. I was diagnosed with high blood pressure and high cholesterol and started taking medication ten years ago. To top it off, I was also diagnosed with depression. The idea that I would have to suffer like this for the rest of my life gave me anxiety. My career was at stake. I was frequently calling in sick and inconsistent with my quality of work. I watched as my colleagues got promoted within the company as I was essentially left behind.

Luckily, at the age of 55, my friend referred me to a Family Health Advocacy doctor who is a functional medicine practitioner. I followed their recommendations and improved my nutrition by making practical changes. I was given guidance on exactly what to eat and not eat. It was explained to me why and how certain foods serve my body well and their benefits. With accountability and a better understanding of how my body works, I started to see changes after week one. I found making changes to my food choices to be simple. Within four weeks, I had more energy and had lost 15 pounds. Of course, with the weight loss and feeling the energy I desperately craved, my mood changed. I could see my relationship with my husband start to strengthen. We started to become more active together and enjoyed each other's company on evening walks. My entire family embraced the change in my food lifestyle. We no longer had pop, chips, chocolate, sugary cereals, or granola bars in our kitchen cupboards. My counter and fridge came to life with the color of fresh foods. One year after I started the program, I had lost 58 lbs and I was still losing weight. Last weekend my entire family went on a ski trip. This would have once been a distant unreachable dream, and now I feel like I'm living again.

Without my friend's help, I would still be in that dark place. I am grateful he pointed me in the right direction. By giving me guidance and a personalized plan that actually worked, my functional medicine practitioner brought me back to life.

Remove Bad Fats/Add Good Fats

Fat has a bad reputation – not all fat is bad! Good fats have many health benefits and we need them in our diet. Good fats deliver fat-soluble vitamins to our body, support metabolism, cell communication, immune function, and hormone regulation. Good fats are important for proper brain function, decreasing symptoms of depression, and improving memory.

Bad fats, such as hydrogenated and partially hydrogenated fats, also known as trans fats, cause cellular congestion and inflammation. There is a strong link between bad fats and heart disease and diabetes, which are two of the many chronic diseases due to inflammation. Bad fats cause cellular congestion and oxidative stress to the cells, resulting in the development of symptoms associated with widespread inflammation, chronic fatigue syndrome, and fibromyalgia. Bad fats result in decreased nerve transmission and decreased focus, memory, and brain function.

If they are so bad for us, why are we consuming them? Just like refined and processed grains, they are cheaper and have a longer shelf life and are therefore used in many packaged foods. As a result, most people are consuming too much omega 6 and trans-fat and not enough omega 3. There is a ratio imbalance.

Most people eat a lot of trans fat without even realizing it. The obvious bad fat foods are fried and battered, so many of us know to stay away from them, but the majority of our bad fat intake is hidden. Most people look at the big square label on the side or back of a food box titled Nutrition Facts. As we mentioned earlier, this part of the label can be misleading. If the amount of trans fat in one serving size of that item contains less than 0.5 grams of trans fat, the product can be labeled "zero percent" trans-fat. The trick of the industry is to decrease the serving size so that they can manipulate the label to look like a cleaner product than it is.

It is essential to read beyond the Nutrition Facts and dig deep into the ingredient list when grocery shopping in order to find the hidden sources. Look for the words "partially hydrogenated" in the ingredients list. If you see those words, then the product contains bad fats.

Trans-fats are used to make liquid vegetable oils more solid (think of the difference between canola oil and margarine) which increases shelf-life and helps maintain the perceived freshness of the food for longer. That's why you will find hidden sources of bad fats in packaged foods like crackers, coffee creamers, cookies, chips, doughnuts, some frozen meals, pizza crust, and margarine.

Cooking Tips:

Olive oil turns rancid if heated above 120 deg.
If it smokes, it is rancid!

For Medium heat use:
extra-virgin olive oil
sesame oil,
grapeseed oil,
coconut oil or butter

For high heat or frying only use
coconut oil or grapeseed oil

For baking use
butter,
coconut oil,
sunflower oil,
safflower or olive oil in less than 325 deg.

It's time to increase our *good* fat intake! Good fats are essential for our health, and yet they are the number one nutritional deficiency in North America. If you are looking to heal and decrease inflammation, crank up your essential fatty acid intake by eating:

- Avocados
- Coconut oil
- Olive oil
- Flax seeds
- Fish
- Meat
- Nuts and seeds

Meat contains many nutrients and amino acids which are beneficial to healing fibromyalgia. If you are a meat-eater, it's important to consume meat only from quality sources, so look for grass fed, pasture-raised, organic, free-roaming, and hormone and antibiotic free. Meat from quality sources contains good fats in the ideal ratio. Commercially raised animals are grain fed, which means they are fed food that they don't naturally eat. Grain-fed animals have an altered fatty acid ratio and as a result, saturated fats become bad fats.

Grass-fed and pasture-raised animals contain essential fatty acids like arachidonic acid, conjugated linoleic acid (CLA), and a proper omega 3-6 ratio. CLA is great for people with fibromyalgia because it helps decrease fat stores that accumulate as a result of the inability to exercise, as well as improves muscle mass.

Omega 3 has a powerful anti-inflammatory action which makes it the most common supplement for fibromyalgia patients. When the omega 3-6 ratio is out of balance and there is more omega 6, it can result in increased inflammation and pain.

Quality meat also contains other important nutrients, like Vitamin B12. Deficiency may appear similar to those symptoms of fibromyalgia: dizziness, numbness, brain fog, fatigue, weakness, anxiety/depression, aches and pains, digestive issues, decreased coordination, and difficulty with balance. A simple blood test can identify a deficiency. A B12 supplement is one of the solutions to deficiency.

Creatine, a nutrient found in meat and fish, helps with muscle function which is crucial when dealing with fibromyalgia. Zinc is found in a variety of foods, like meat, seafood, beans, seeds, lentils, and peas. It improves cognition and helps with "brain fog," and improves your mood and immune system. Zinc is important because it is also on the anti-inflammatory team. Meats are rich in selenium which also helps decrease inflammation, reduce free radicals and oxidative stress while increasing blood flow and circulation.

The many benefits of eating quality meat can be outweighed if the meat is actually highly processed commercial grade. Not only are commercially raised animals being fed foods they don't naturally eat, they are also given antibiotics in order to stay disease-free in the cramped unsanitary pens they live in. These antibiotics are found in the meat. Hormones are given to commercially raised animals to help fatten them up, and these hormones can also stay in the meat and affect our own hormones.

Avoid processed meats as well, as they often contain preservatives like sodium nitrite and salt which aggravates pain and swelling. The bottom line: You aren't just what you eat…you are what you're eating ate. Choose your meats wisely. Meat is at the top of the food chain and worth investing in.

Fish

Fish is an excellent source of essential fatty acid. Research links fibromyalgia to high levels of mercury, so make sure you choose fish with lower levels. Wild fish also typically have lower mercury levels and a better omega 3-6 ratio than farmed fish.

Low-Mercury – Sardines, tilapia, salmon, flounder, herring

Moderate-Mercury – Cod, haddock, bluefish, freshwater bass, sea bass

High-Mercury – Albacore tuna, marlin, orange roughy, tuna, swordfish, shark, bluefin tuna

Toxic – Crab, lobster, mussels, oysters, scallops, and shrimp are bottom-feeding scavengers, which means they contain all sorts of things you wouldn't want to be putting in your body.

Coconut Oil

Coconut oil is great for fibromyalgia as it contains a high level of a medium chain fatty acid called laurate (lauric acid), which your body uses for energy. It is also a great supplement for intestinal disorders, which are common symptoms of fibromyalgia.

Caffeine

Caffeine is the world's most commonly consumed drug. It is addictive, yet legal. It gives people an energy boost when needed and has an effect that lasts for hours. As a result, over-consumption of caffeine is an epidemic. It's tempting for a lot of people with fibromyalgia to fight symptoms like fatigue with a steady dose of caffeine from soft drinks or coffee. Some people are more sensitive than others to the effects of caffeine. For some, consuming as little as a few sips of coffee may lead to insomnia, sweating, nervousness, restlessness, irritability, an upset stomach, increased heart rate, and even muscle twitching.

Reports show that caffeine has an effect on bone mass and increases fracture risks. Caffeine has no nutritional value. When consuming caffeine even hours before bed, you can interfere with your ability to get restful sleep. This is a roadblock for fibromyalgia sufferers because quality sleep is essential in minimizing painful symptoms. Caffeine's direct effect on the brain may exacerbate symptoms of depression, anxiety, or restlessness, which are commonly experienced amongst fibromyalgia sufferers. Caffeine should be limited or avoided altogether.

Aspartame and Artificial Sweetener

Studies indicate that food additives impact fibromyalgia. Food additives, the most common of which is aspartame, cause a chemical reaction that triggers pain.

Aspartame is often used to add flavor. It's a sugar substitute used in foods and beverages, and in many products labeled "diet" or "sugar-free." It is often sold under the brand names NutraSweet and Equal.

The safety of aspartame and artificial sweeteners is controversial. While some studies have reported that it is safe for human consumption, other reports link aspartame to cancer, thyroid suppression, chronic pain, and fibromyalgia. In a 2010 article published in *Clinical and Experimental Rheumatology*, individuals discontinued aspartame consumption and their fibromyalgia symptoms abated and did not recur. Although the numbers in this article are not staggering, the potential benefit of eliminating aspartame from your diet makes it worthwhile, especially since the benefit of keeping it in your diet is non-existent.

Water

Coffee, tea, and soda are not thirst quenching. In fact, they're all diuretics, which means they contribute to dehydration and require you to drink more water. Thirst, fatigue, irritability, headache, feeling faint and dizzy, urine that is dark and strong smelling…. these are all signs you are probably dehydrated.

Your body weight is made up of sixty percent water, and seventy-five percent of muscles are comprised of water. Water intake is vital for proper function and health. You have probably read that, as a general rule, you should consume eight eight-ounce glasses of water a day. It's referred to as the 8X8 rule. 8X8 is a start! However, everybody is different and has different requirements. Sweating, breathing, offsetting the drinking of diuretics, and getting rid of waste in your system requires more water intake. When demands are high, you lose more fluid than you take in and become dehydrated. Adjust your water intake depending on your workout schedule, or if you are living in a hot climate since you expel water when you sweat.

Recommended water intake can be much more individualized. There are a lot of different ways to calculate how much water you should consume. Although the calculations may vary slightly, they all drive home the undebatable fact that water is essential for good health.

Water helps you stay healthy and energized. It also:

- Controls your body temperature
- Aids digestion
- Carries nutrients around your body
- Cushions organs and joints
- Gets rid of waste
- Keeps your bowels regular
- Aids in weight loss

Tips to Increase Water Intake

Use these tips to help you increase your water intake and stay hydrated!

1. Drink two cups of water before every meal, even breakfast! We often think that we are hungrier than we are because we confuse hunger with dehydration. Drinking before a meal will curb your appetite and help you with portion control.

2. Keep a water container handy at all times. We both have water containers we use in our treatment rooms at the office. Our team ensures that our water containers are full before our shift of seeing patients begins. They refill the containers at least twice during a three-hour shift. Water consumption is so important, however often forgotten about until signs of dehydration set in. Not everyone has a team encouraging them to drink water and refilling their container throughout the day. Find a container you love and set a goal for how many refills you will need during that day.

3. Flavor! We absolutely love water. Some people don't. Have no fear, infusion is near! Add fruit like strawberries, watermelon, lemon, limes, cucumber, and berries to make your water more exciting to drink. Be creative and have fun. Do not add artificial flavorings.

4. Start the day with a large glass of water and end the day with a small glass of water. We drink a glass before bed each night. We also put a glass next to the bed to quench thirst in the middle of the night or first thing in the morning.

5. Fizz or carbonation can cause some digestive issues like heartburn, gas, and irritate ulcers. Carbonation also causes a change in bone density. Drinking carbonated water should be done in

moderation and as an alternative to the soda, coffee, tea, and beverages you are looking to wean off of.

Dairy

Many fibromyalgia sufferers have lactose sensitivities. Digestive symptoms resulting from intolerance to lactose include bloating, gas, pain, and cramping. Flare-ups of other fibromyalgia symptoms may also be related to dairy consumption. Intolerance levels can vary from mild sensitivities to severe reactions. If you have a suspicion that you may be intolerant to lactose, eliminate dairy from your diet for six weeks and note any changes and improvements in your health.

There are many lactose-free dairy options and alternatives, such as coconut and almond milk, available in most grocery stores. Avoid fat-free options as that often means sugar has been added. Sugar can increase inflammation and aggravate symptoms.

If you are confident you are not lactose intolerant, we recommend you stick to organic dairy products.

Fruit

Fruit contains many essential vitamins, minerals, fiber, and antioxidants, but many people consume too much fruit and suffer from high sugar intakes that they aren't even aware of. You need to give your body a break from the insulin and leptin spikes and eliminate sugar, even fructose from fruit sources. Don't forget, sugar has been causing inflammation, and inflammation is the initiating cause of chronic disease and pain because it disrupts hormonal signaling throughout the body.

When you are in a healing mode, it's important to remember not all fruit is created equal. Some fruits have a high glycemic index and are high in acidity. When focused on healing, you want to minimize sugar spikes by sticking to low glycemic index foods in order to help regulate leptin and insulin levels. While placing emphasis on reducing widespread inflammation in the body, stick to eating fruit in the morning and mid-day. Berries are a great fruit source, rich in anti- inflammatory, antioxidant, and anti-aging properties. Berries also have a low glycemic index load. Other low glycemic index fruits include:

Blueberries	Oranges	Apricots
Strawberries	Lemon/Lime	Nectarines
Raspberries	Grapes	Plums
Blackberries	Kiwi	Passionfruit
Pears	Cherries	Melons

Grapefruit	Apples	Pomegranates
Dates	Peaches	Avocados

Remember to choose fresh fruits, in-season and organic when possible.

Below is a list of fruits to eat sparingly. All of these fruits are broken down into categories based on the speed at which your body metabolizes them and their effect on leptin and insulin hormones.

Fruit to Eat Sparingly

- Banana
- Mango
- Papaya
- Pineapple
- Watermelon

MSG

Monosodium Glutamate, or MSG, is added to many foods as a flavoring agent or enhancer, and it also prolongs shelf life. MSG is often used in canned or frozen foods, processed meats, boxed snacks, and fast foods. MSG is a compound of sodium – basic table salt – and glutamate, which is a naturally occurring amino acid found in foods like tomatoes, walnuts, and cheese. Some people have sensitivities to MSG that manifest as headaches, and it can also increase sensitivity to pain. Studies have shown a decrease of pain symptoms in fibromyalgia patients within months of eliminating MSG from their diet.

When grocery shopping, check the label for MSG or Monosodium glutamate. There are various names for MSG and other ingredients that have a high MSG content but aren't required to say so.

Look out for these ingredients on food labels:

Glutamic Acid (E 620)	Autolyzed protein	Spices
Glutamate (E 621-625)	Plant or textured protein	Yeast extract
Anything hydrolyzed	Hydrolyzed vegetable protein	Natural flavoring
Caseinate	Gelatin	

The best way to avoid food additives is to eat foods from the earth and stay away from packaged, processed foods.

Intermittent Fasting

Intermittent fasting is gaining popularity in the health and fitness world because of the beneficial physiological effects. Humans have used fasting methods for thousands of years for many reasons, including food availability, religious observances, and sickness. Intermittent fasting involves alternating cycles of fasting and eating. The focus lies on *when* you eat rather than *what* you eat. Combine the two and the results are even better!

There are many different intermittent fasting methods but all of them divide the week into fasting periods and eating periods. While you are sleeping, you are fasting. Intermittent fasting can be as simple as extending that fast a little longer by skipping breakfast, eating your first meal a little later in the day, or finishing your dinner earlier in the evening.

The most popular intermittent fasting method is the 16/8, restricting your eating window to eight hours and the fasting window to sixteen hours. Many people report they have increased levels of energy during the fasting periods.

Intermittent fasting is easier than most people might assume, which is one of the reasons why it's gaining popularity. Although popular as a weight loss method, there are many people who fast for general wellness, including metabolic health and disease prevention.

Numerous studies underline the health benefits of fasting, including:

1. Cellular repair
2. Hormone regulation
3. Increased metabolism
4. Weight loss
5. Reduced insulin resistance

6. Decreased risk of type 2 diabetes
7. Reduced oxidative stress and inflammation
8. Reduced blood pressure
9. Reduced cholesterol
10. Decreased risk of cancer
11. Improved brain function
12. Extended lifespan

Research has also demonstrated that intermittent fasting improves the symptoms of fibromyalgia.

Paula's Story

I was overweight and feeling constantly tired. I really did not feel good about myself at all. I weighed 141 pounds at 5'3. I disliked looking at myself in the mirror and just felt embarrassed. Not being very tall made my weight gain extremely noticeable and quite frankly it was uncomfortable for me both physically and socially. I was tired and feeling sluggish. Unfortunately, I caught myself eating more and more and I was becoming less active. I was eating to feel better emotionally. The more I ate, the more I wanted to eat. I was eating throughout the day. It was a vicious cycle. I thought eating three times a day, plus snacks, was the better way to stay healthy and maintain an appropriate weight for my height, but it wasn't helping me.

I initially started intermittent fasting without actually intending to do so. I am a teacher and I work in a high-needs busy classroom. I learned more about intermittent fasting and started to make better food choices. I lost 16 pounds and now weigh 125 pounds. I feel better about myself and I don't feel like I need to eat all the time. I eat <u>when</u> and <u>if</u> I'm hungry but it's usually in the evenings. I feel energized and more alive.

Orlando's Story

Prior to starting intermittent fasting, I had gotten up to 289 lbs standing at nearly 5'10". That is a lot of weight! I found that in my late 30s and early 40s, I was going to the gym for four hours at a time and I wasn't really losing weight. I would just bulk up with muscle. My metabolism was slow.

The extra weight was really tiring me out and making me feel exhausted all the time. I suffered from various strains, including a knee injury that made me slow down at the gym and the extra weight gain began. That is when the doctors taught me about intermittent fasting. Everything made sense to me. Being busy at work, making time to meal prep, shop, cook, and eat became stressful. Once I started the intermittent fasting, I found that I had much more time on my hands and less stress. Instead of feeling heavy at the end of my 9 to 5 work day, I actually felt lighter and had more energy. I have now refined what I eat in the eating window and the results keep coming.

In four months, I had lost 45 lbs. In a full calendar year, I had lost 65 lbs. I feel much better. My health has improved. I have more energy later in the day, sleep better, and feel stronger. I get sick less often. Dr. Morgan and Dr. Casey have helped me deal with the damage I had done to my body over the many years of neglect. I definitely get more done in my day, my mind works better, I feel better and have more energy. Thanks to Dr. Morgan, Dr. Casey, and intermittent fasting. It is a new way of life!

Chapter Recap: Top Foods to Avoid

- Sugar
- Bad Fats
- Processed grains
- Caffeine
- Aspartame & Artificial Sweeteners
- Gluten
- Dairy
- MSG

In summary, drastically reduce sugar intake, limit grain consumption and choose whole or sprouted grains, and focus on low glycemic index foods. Revisit the nutrition section often to remind yourself of what to eat and why.

Mmmm

Here are just a few of the endless options for healthy meals. It makes sense to wrap up a chapter on nutrition by inspiring your taste buds! For recipes and more meal ideas, visit familyhealthadvocacy.com.

Breakfast Ideas
- Scrambled egg and avocado
- Oatmeal
- Banana and nut butter on whole grain toast
- Protein powder smoothie
- Quinoa fruit salad
- Black bean and egg burrito

Lunch & Snack Ideas
- Hardboiled egg
- Apple with nut butter
- Rice cake with nut butter
- Kale or zucchini chips
- Hummus and veggies (carrots, celery, zucchini, cherry tomatoes, broccoli, cauliflower)
- Nuts

Dinner Ideas
- Wild caught salmon with mashed cauliflower
- Free range chicken with asparagus
- Zucchini noodles with choice of vegetables
- Lettuce wrap tacos
- Homemade stew/soup

SUPPLEMENTS

The word supplement is often misunderstood as a replacement for something. Some people think that if they take vitamins, they don't have to choose healthy food sources or make changes to their lifestyle. However, the definition of supplement is "something that completes or enhances something else when added to it." The best way to heal is to have a healthy diet and lifestyle, and then take supplements to enhance the solid foundation you have laid.

Vitamin D

Studies have shown that people who suffer from fibromyalgia have lower vitamin D levels. This is no surprise, as vitamin D insufficiency affects approximately fifty percent of the population worldwide.

Vitamin D3 is made when the skin is exposed to the sun's ultraviolet rays, but it is extremely difficult to get sufficient amounts naturally, especially in colder climates. Skin tone affects the amount of D3 one can absorb from the sun: it's more readily absorbed in lighter skin tones, while darker tones and elderly people require three to five times longer exposure.

Vitamin D deficiency is linked to a number of diseases including cancer, poor mitochondrial function, musculoskeletal pain, and weakness. Increasing vitamin D3 levels improves immune function, lowers inflammation, and helps with the absorption of phosphate and calcium in the gastrointestinal tract, which is necessary for bone health and improved immune function.

Here are some more benefits of Vitamin D:

1. Protects against colds and flu
2. Good for your teeth, bones, and helps your muscles, nerves, and immune system work better
3. High doses of Vitamin D (20,000 or 40,000 IU weekly) for one year can improve symptoms of depression
4. Lowers pain levels

Here are the vitamin D intake levels recommended for patients at risk for vitamin D deficiency. These numbers are taken from the Endocrine Practice Guidelines Committee. IU= International Units.

- Infants: 400–1,000 IU/day (upper limit: 2,000)
- Children 1 -18 years: 600-1,000 IUs/day (upper limit 4,000)
- Adults: 19 +: 1,500-2,000 IU's/day (upper limit 10,000)

A simple blood test will determine if you are vitamin D deficient. A month after you begin supplementation, we recommend you get your vitamin D levels tested again to determine if your level is sufficient. In addition to supplementation and the sun, you can also get Vitamin D from foods like eggs, fatty fish like salmon and mackerel, and fortified dairy products.

Fatty Acids:
Omega Supplementation

Omega fatty acids are another one of the supplements we commonly recommend. Essential fatty acids are one of the most common nutritional deficiencies in North America, and EPA (eicosapentaenoic acid) and DHA (docosa-hexaenoic acid) are the best sources. They are called essential fatty acids because our body does not produce them naturally. The optimal diet would include intake of omega 6 and omega 3 at a ratio of 2:1, but most North American diets are closer to 20:1.

Omega supplements must be kept cool to avoid oxidation damage. Omega-3 fatty acids are often taken in the form of fish oil or flaxseed oil. Fish, flax, krill or algae oil are all good sources of 'good fats.'

Good fats decrease inflammation, which is linked to many diseases including, of course, fibromyalgia. As a result, good fats have been associated with reducing incidence of cancer, dementia, arthritis, asthma, allergies, eczema, digestive disease, and joint pain. They also improve blood pressure, nerve conduction, mood and brain function, hormone regulation, and are important for normal growth and development. Dietary omega-3 fatty acids are in several foods, including:

- Seaweed
- Algae
- Walnuts
- Canola and hemp seed oils
- Fatty fish (salmon, tuna, herring, sardines, anchovies)
- Egg yolk
- Soybeans (careful of GMO)
- Grass-fed beef
- Flaxseeds and flaxseed oil

Be aware of mercury or lead contamination and be conscious of what type of fish is used and where it is sourced from. This is why good-quality supplementation from a provider you trust is essential.

Supplementation Tips

There are different forms of omega supplements, including pure fish oil and processed fish oil. The EPA and DHA percentage will vary depending on the type and source of oil. Therefore, it's best to follow recommendations given on the packaging of each specific supplement. Know what your omega supplement contains. Like any other product, we recommend you look at the label on the back of the product and evaluate the EPA and DHA percentage. Natural pure fish oil usually consists of no more than thirty percent EPA and DHA, which means seventy percent is other fats designed to help with absorption.

Processed fish oil is usually cleaned of contaminants such as mercury. These oils often contain EPA and DHA levels of fifty to ninety percent. It is best to take these supplements with a fat-containing meal to aid in the absorption of omega-3s. Regardless of your supplement choice, keep in mind that omegas are perishable. Note the expiration date and check to see if the oil has gone rancid by smelling it periodically. A quality vegetarian and vegan option is algae supplementation.

Magnesium

Magnesium is a mineral that plays an important role in many systems of the body. It is most known for its role in keeping the heart healthy, blood pressure normal, and bones strong. Magnesium deficiency is becoming more and more common and supplementation has very few risks of side effects. Those who are deficient in magnesium are likely to have elevated inflammation markers, so it is no surprise that magnesium deficiency is common in women with fibromyalgia. Magnesium is concentrated in the mitochondria of cells, so when magnesium levels are low, energy cannot be metabolized. Magnesium is essential for proper muscle function and nerve transmission.

Magnesium deficiency has become more common as a result of the depletion of magnesium in our soil, resulting in a lowered amount in crops and food. On top of that is poor nutrition and food choices which lack magnesium. Magnesium is also depleted with consumption of caffeinated beverages like soda, coffee, and tea, which all produce a diuretic effect and an increased loss of the mineral through urine. Damage to the intestinal tract from prescription drugs along with digestive disorders also results in malabsorption of magnesium and other minerals and nutrients in the gut. Calcium supplementation is common in North America but can lead to magnesium deficiency as well.

Another contributing factor to magnesium deficiency is chronic stress, which results in a constant release of neurotransmitters and the hormone cortisol (the "stress hormone") which depletes magnesium.

Testing for magnesium deficiency is commonly done by measuring concentrations in the blood, saliva, and urine. However, assessing magnesium levels through a general blood test is difficult and challenges accuracy, resulting in misleading results. This is because most magnesium resides in the bones and cells. A more accurate and less common test used for magnesium deficiency is by measuring the Red Blood Cell (RBC) test. When your body is low in magnesium, it will take what it needs from the cells, including RBCs.

Magnesium supplementation is very safe, and many doctors will suggest supplementation based on health history and symptoms without performing a test.

Magnesium supplements are most common in pill form, but magnesium is transdermal, meaning it can be rapidly absorbed through your skin. Gels, creams, and oils that contain magnesium are available, and Epsom salts baths also help. It is commonly recommended to start with 350 mg/day when supplementing with magnesium. If you take too much, a potential side effect is diarrhea.

Supplementing regularly in combination with eating magnesium-rich foods is a wise and simple way to combat deficiency. Dietary sources include black-eyed peas, legumes, Swiss chard, avocado, broccoli, squash, pumpkin seeds, cashews, almonds, whole grains such as brown rice, and fish.

Magnesium supplementation has shown to improve immune function and decrease inflammation and pain, both of which are symptoms of fibromyalgia.

Coenzyme Q10

COQ10 is a powerful natural antioxidant produced by the body, but production decreases with age, making supplementation even more important as we get older. Prescription drugs such as statins or beta blockers can decrease COQ10 levels by up to forty percent, so supplementing is important to compensate for this loss. Athletes and fitness enthusiasts commonly take a COQ10 supplement as strenuous exercise can further decrease levels.

COQ10 has gained a lot of recognition over the past ten years as studies have associated decreased levels of COQ10 with a wide variety of diseases, including heart conditions, blood sugar regulation problems, fatigue, brain fog, joint pain, muscle stiffness, headaches, difficulty with balance and coordination, stomach ulcers, and more.

COQ10 supplementation is of special interest to the fibromyalgia community. A 2009 study showed that nearly half (44.8 percent) of patients with chronic fatigue syndrome and fibromyalgia had COQ10 deficiency.

COQ10 inhibits oxidation and is important in 95 percent of all ATP production in the mitochondria. It also helps initiate the cell death of mutated or damaged cells. With evidence showing that mitochondrial dysfunction and oxidative stress likely play a role in fibromyalgia, it's not a surprise that COQ10 supplementation is more commonly used and can significantly improve clinical symptoms of fibromyalgia.

Studies are also showing other common benefits of COQ10:

- Decreases inflammation
- Reduces pain
- Reduces fatigue
- Reduces muscles weakness
- Reduces headaches
- Increases immune function
- Increases serotonin levels and improves mood
- Regenerates glutathione

COQ10 is found in food sources like seafood, organic meats such as liver and hearts, and is present in smaller amounts in vegetarian options such as broccoli, nuts, and seeds. However, it would be extremely difficult to achieve proper levels without supplementation.

Average recommended supplementation is 150-200mg /day. Therapeutic doses can be as high as 1,000mg /day depending on the individual condition. Keep in mind that different supplement brands might have different ingredients and strengths. Follow the instructions on the bottle unless otherwise instructed by your healthcare practitioner.

When taken as a supplement on its own, choose the soft gel ubiquinol form of COQ10, as it has greater antioxidant efficiency than the cheaper ubiquinone form. However, most COQ10 supplements are a combination of both.

Multivitamin

Good-quality, whole-food multivitamins are the foundation to supplementation. Everyone in your family should be taking a multivitamin. It's a daily guarantee to ensure your body gets the vitamins, minerals, and essential nutrients it needs.

It's important to note that not all vitamins are created equal. In fact, some can do more harm than good. If you find your vitamins on the shelf of the grocery store or drugstore, they are most likely synthetic products with a low level of absorption resulting in little to no benefit to the body. Some of these supplements even contain fillers, colors, preservatives, and ingredients you want to avoid. When we were kids, a lot of our friends were taking cartoon-themed chewable vitamins and popping them like candy. When you look at the ingredient list, you can see that they are hardly better than candy! These multivitamins are prime examples of supplements to stay away from.

Whole food multivitamins are made from real foods, and therefore digest and absorb properly and become nutrients your body can use. It can be daunting to choose which multivitamin is best for you, so we recommend getting yours from a trusted source. Visit a natural food or supplement store where there is someone you can talk to about quality and the ingredients. Do your research on the company and their brand.

Check into the online community for more information on our best recommendations and what we use personally.

You may be wondering if a healthy nutrition plan negates the need for a daily multivitamin. Our short answer is no. Although whole foods offer good sources of vitamins, the majority of even healthy diets are nutrient deficient. Modern fast-paced agriculture practices, nutrient-deficient soils, genetic modification, pesticides, food travel time, food processing (both commercially and at home) and additives are reasons why. Embracing a high-quality multivitamin into your daily routine is a good idea for everyone.

Probiotics

Probiotics are crucial to healing digestive problems associated with fibromyalgia. They are found naturally in foods like yogurt, but there is an insufficient amount to be of therapeutic effect. Probiotic supplements come in various forms: capsules, powder, and a concentrated yogurt found in the natural food store.

Probiotics help with proper function of the gastrointestinal tract, and up to seventy percent of our immune system is located in our digestive tract! In addition, they have notable benefits in treating mental illness and neurological disorders.

Choose a strong probiotic that can withstand the acidity of the digestive tract and re-establishes "friendly" bacteria in your gut. The goal is to bring the levels of "good" and "bad" bacteria back into balance.

Probiotics are live healthy bacteria so it's important to store them in the fridge after opening. Probiotics help reduce yeast when there is overgrowth and are commonly used to alleviate symptoms of irritable bowel syndrome and acid reflux. A 2008 study revealed a relationship between the decrease of gut flora and the increase of symptoms of fibromyalgia.

If bacteria are natural in our body, how did they get out of balance in the first place?

1. Over-sterilization of foods
2. Overuse of antibiotics
3. Overconsumption of grains and sugar
4. Fluoride and chlorine in water kill healthy bacteria
5. Lack of digestive enzymes as we age

You can see why this is such an important supplement to be taken daily. In addition to probiotics, we also regularly consume organic fermented foods like kimchi, kefir, and sauerkraut. Although we recommend probiotics on a daily basis for everyone, if you are skeptical or want to just test the waters, we suggest a two-month trial.

Digestive Enzymes

Digestive enzymes are proteins that facilitate the breakdown of food and help convert food into energy. We strive to eat proper foods, improve our nutrition, and take supplements, but what's the point if our bodies aren't absorbing all these nutrients properly? Digestive enzymes are a game changer.

We are both around forty years old and can observe our bodies aging – they aren't producing and functioning like they did twenty years ago. One of the things our bodies produce less of as we age are digestive enzymes, making it more difficult to break down fats and carbohydrates. That's why you commonly hear people say digestion slows down with age.

I'm sure you have experienced those meals where you feel sluggish and still full hours later, having a hard time to get going for the rest of the day. It's annoying!

Taking digestive enzymes with your meal improves digestion and prevents food from remaining in your stomach for too long, which would create irritation of the intestinal lining, irritable bowel, and GERD. If the lining becomes porous, food particles can penetrate the wall and enter the bloodstream, inciting an inflammatory reaction.

Because we also produce less stomach acid as we get older, it's important to take a digestive enzyme that contains betaine hydrochloric acid, unless you have an ulcer. If this is the case, stick to a supplement that only includes pancreatic enzymes.

Richard's Story

I'm 28 years old and have been working as a nurse for two years. In addition to all of my pain, I also experienced serious digestive problems that resulted in frequent trips to the hospital. Eating and drinking would cause excruciating pain. I was extremely underweight and malnourished. I was unable to maintain focus and would have mood swings. I knew I had to do something but everything I was trying wasn't working. I had become skeptical about everything.

Since starting this program, my health has improved greatly. I followed the nutrition and exercise plan and corrected the alignment of my spine and pelvis, reducing stress on the nerves to my digestive organs. My mood is so much better and I now experience a sense of ease and peace. I look better too, as I maintain a healthy weight. I absolutely love this lifestyle and plan to keep it up. I feel like a better person overall! I recommend this program because the doctors are great at coaching you to help you improve your overall health.

Turmeric/Curcumin

Turmeric is a plant originating in India that is ground into an orange-colored spice; curcumin is the active ingredient. Curcumin is a strong antioxidant, a powerful anti-inflammatory, and effective painkiller. It has been reported that curcumin is more effective than conventional painkillers and has none of the contraindications. Curcumin also helps balance chemicals in the brain, resulting in improved cognition, memory, hormone regulation, sleep, and energy levels. Curcumin reduces inflammation and therefore reduces symptoms of rheumatism, irritable bowel syndrome, autoimmune and inflammatory diseases. It also improves and regulates immune function as it acts as an antimicrobial, terminating viral infections. It's also been shown to alleviate symptoms of depression and anxiety.

Add fresh or ground turmeric to soups and stews, smoothies, or even baking. Turmeric also comes as a supplement in capsule form to be taken with meals. The suggested amount is 1000-2000 mg daily, or as symptoms suggest.

Melatonin

Melatonin is a hormone that's naturally produced by the pineal gland in the brain. Proper secretion of this hormone is responsible for regulating other hormones, helping you fall asleep and regulating your sleep patterns. Low melatonin levels are associated with inadequate sleep, poor memory and cognition, digestive issues, low metabolism, and other symptoms associated with fibromyalgia. In this digital age, our brains are over-stimulated. Most people aren't getting enough sleep and our bodies aren't producing enough melatonin. Blood pressure medications (beta-blockers) will also inhibit melatonin secretion. Many studies have demonstrated that melatonin is effective in reducing pain in fibromyalgia sufferers.

The recommended dosage is 1 to 10mg in the evening. We suggest starting with a small dose.

SAMe (S-adenosylmethionine)

SAMe is a naturally occurring molecule in our bodies which decreases with age. It can be recommended as a supplement for fibromyalgia patients experiencing anxiety and difficulty sleeping. This supplement is most commonly taken orally at 600 mg-1600mg/day. It's been shown to increase serotonin, norepinephrine, and dopamine levels, and reduce pain, inflammation, and depression. It is also a great detoxifier as it increases the synthesis of glutathione. Some side effects include stomach upset and nausea, so it's important to start with a low dose to see how it affects you.

5-HTP – 5 Hydroxy-Tryptophan

Low serotonin levels have long been linked to fibromyalgia. Serotonin is a neurotransmitter that regulates appetite, melatonin production, mood, and cognition. 5-HTP is a precursor to serotonin but requires vitamin B6 for its conversion. Studies have shown that 5-HTP improves fibromyalgia symptoms, decreasing widespread pain and its severity, reducing sleeplessness and headaches.

A common recommendation for dosage of supplementation is 100mg 3 times/day orally (and up to 1000 mg).

Stomach upset is a potential side effect and 5-HTP should not be taken with antidepressants or monoamine oxidase inhibitors.

D-Ribose

D-Ribose is a form of sugar and is naturally produced by your cells. The mitochondria use D-ribose to produce ATP energy which is great for combatting fibromyalgia and chronic fatigue syndrome symptoms of fatigue, pain, and muscle weakness.

A frequently suggested dose is 5mg two or three times per day. Some potential side effects include stomach upset and nausea, headaches, and low blood sugar.

Chlorella

Chlorella is freshwater algae containing vitamins, minerals, enzymes, amino acids, and chlorophyll. It is a powerful antioxidant and boosts the immune system by increasing good intestinal bacteria, also improving digestion. Chlorella has been shown to reduce pain and anxiety and improve sleep. It can also alleviate inflammation of the large intestine.

Spirulina

Spirulina is a blue-green alga that's a cousin to chlorophyll. Spirulina is a superfood plant source of protein, minerals, vitamins like calcium and iron, and antioxidants. Spirulina has a powerful anti-inflammatory effect and acts as an immunity booster. People notice a myriad of benefits from its anti-inflammatory properties including improvements in cholesterol levels, blood pressure, energy levels, and pain relief.

Additional Supplements

Here is a list of additional supplements shown to be beneficial for people suffering from chronic pain and fibromyalgia. We will go into more detail about these supplements in our online community.

Greens Powder – Filled with vitamins, minerals, and antioxidants. Greens boost immune function and reduce inflammation.

Vitamin K – Known for its blood clotting and bone strengthening properties, it also reduces overall fibromyalgia symptoms, particularly pain.

Vitamin E – An antioxidant. According to a small 2015 study, women with fibromyalgia who consumed less vitamin E had higher severity of symptoms. The study suggests that vitamin E may have an impact on quality of life.

Vitamin C – Also known as L-ascorbic acid/ascorbate. It is an antioxidant, reducing free radical damage. Vitamin C protects and maintains cellular health, boosts metabolism, and helps immune function. It is important in promoting healthy connective tissue and organs. Vitamin C is needed for the biosynthesis of collagen, which is a vital element of the healing process. It has been shown that combining Vitamin C and E with exercise can reduce oxidative stress in fibromyalgia patients.

AMPK (5-adenosine monophosphate-activated protein kinase) – An enzyme found naturally throughout the body; it regulates cellular energy levels. Activated AMPK helps fat and blood sugar burning and converts it into energy in the mitochondria. It is believed that AMPK is inactive or under-activated in people with fibromyalgia resulting in lower energy production. AMPK helps fight against chronic pain and inflammation.

Several nutrients help restore the AMPK activation including Coenzyme Q10, Resveratrol, omega-3 and curcumin.

Taurine – An amino acid and building block of protein. Taurine has been shown to be low in many fibromyalgia patients. Deficiency in taurine may result in vision problems, hypertension or high cholesterol, mood changes, depression, anxiety, weight gain, problems with endurance, and recovery after activity.

Garlic – Known for its antibiotic properties, garlic has been used for generations as a healthy alternative when fighting infections and viruses. Many people with fibromyalgia suffer from chronic infections and have experienced garlic's remarkable ability to stimulate the immune system. Garlic also has powerful anti-inflammatory properties which contribute to pain relief.

L-Arginine – An antioxidant and amino acid that supports the production of nitric oxide, which is typically in low levels in fibromyalgia patients. It promotes healthy blood flow and has been shown to decrease pain symptoms.

L-Citrulline – A non-essential fatty amino acid derived from watermelon, peanuts, soybeans, and kidney beans. Our bodies convert L-Citrulline into L-Arginine to produce nitric oxide. It plays an important role in the urea cycle, which is the process of eliminating toxic by-products from the digestion of protein. L-Citrulline increases heart health, blood flow, and endurance while increasing muscle growth and recovery. It fights free radicals.

Nattokinase – An enzyme extracted from a Japanese food called natto that undergoes a specific fermentation process. Fermenting the soybeans creates healthy bacteria. Nattokinase thins the blood, lowers clotting levels, and has been used to protect against conditions such as stroke, heart attack, muscle spasms, chronic fatigue syndrome, and fibromyalgia.

Red Yeast Rice – A side effect of cholesterol medication is muscle pain. Red yeast rice is a great natural alternative for lowering cholesterol in fibromyalgia patients.

Calcium – Widely known to be important for bone strength, it is also important in muscle contraction. Calcium deficiency can contribute to muscle weakness, cramping, aches and pains, and other symptoms associated with fibromyalgia.

Quercetin – When you think of quercetin, think *red*! Quercetin is commonly found in foods like red grapes, red tomatoes, red raspberries, red wine, red onions, red apples, and also green tea. It's a flavonoid that gives fruits and vegetables their colors. Quercetin is a powerful energy-booster, anti-inflammatory, antioxidant, immunity-booster, and increases glutathione.

Resveratrol – One of the most powerful antioxidants on the planet. It's found in red wine and the skin of grapes. It has strong anti-aging properties and protects organs like the brain and heart. It fights free-radicals and can reduce pain and improve mood.

Green tea – Drinking tea should be an easy addition to your routine and a good way to start your day. Green tea contains polyphenols and theanine.

Polyphenols – These antioxidants reduce oxidative stress, decrease pain and improve quality of life in people with fibromyalgia. High polyphenol foods include berries, cocoa, fruits, tea, and nuts.

L-Theanine – An antioxidant and amino acid found naturally in tea leaves and some mushrooms. It promotes relaxation without making you drowsy. As a result of feeling relaxed, anxiety decreases while alertness, memory, and energy are improved. It also protects brain cells, increases levels of neurotransmitters, dopamine, and norepinephrine, and it lowers activity of neurotransmitter glutamate. Finally, it boosts the production of T-cells in the immune system and helps regulate the sleep-wake cycle.

Poly MVA – Less well known but worth exploring if you are looking deep for answers. Poly MVA (Palladium Alpha-lipoic acid Complex) is an energy-promoting supplement which is a combination of vitamins, minerals, and amino acids. It supports cellular energy production and exerts antioxidant effects.

Selenium – A mineral found in soil, food, and water that is essential for proper immune system function and metabolism. Selenium is most known for its antioxidant properties. Fibromyalgia patients often have low levels of selenium. Food sources that are high in selenium include brazil nuts, seafood, muscle and organ meats, cereals, grains, and dairy products.

The War on Supplements

Millions of North Americans take vitamins and supplements to either achieve or maintain good health. These people swear by the benefits they have experienced using these supplements and do so with very little reason to worry about potential side-effects. There are potential side-effects that can be serious in extremely rare cases and are usually due to over-consumption. Even with all the health benefits and track record of safety, the FDA and many medical doctors constantly berate these supplements, exhorting the public not to use them due to their alleged dangers.

This seems ironic when you consider the FDA stands firmly behind prescription and over-the-counter drugs that can cause people harm even when used properly. Many fibromyalgia sufferers have taken drugs such as NSAIDs in an attempt to ease their symptoms. It still surprises us how many patients come into our clinic who use NSAIDs but are completely unaware of the potential side-effects. These side effects include heart attacks, strokes, high blood pressure, heart failure, stomach bleeds and ulcers, as well as kidney and liver damage.

Digestive problems are a side-effect of NSAID use and also a common symptom of fibromyalgia. Commonly used drugs for digestive issues are known as proton pump inhibitors – an estimated 15 million Americans are on them. These drugs are either prescribed or taken over-the-counter. A serious potential side-effect of these drugs includes increased risk of stroke and heart attack. Many people using these drugs have no clue. Other potential dangers are infections, dementia, kidney damage, and bone fractures. However, the FDA continues to turn a blind eye to these potentially harmful and life-threatening drugs and instead focusing its attention on natural dietary supplements.

Why is this happening? Supplements are natural. They are made up of naturally occurring molecules, and thus cannot be patented. That means there is no money in it for pharmaceutical companies. Surprise! Suggesting pharmaceutical companies are more interested in their profit than your health.

With the FDA sitting comfortably in the back pocket of the pharmaceutical companies, the supplement industry faces strict opposition at every corner. Although supplements on the shelf are approved by the FDA, they are constantly under scrutiny. No amount of research or science in support of natural supplements will gain the acceptance of the FDA due to its relationship with Big Pharma.

AVOID TOXINS

No matter how health conscious you are, you are exposed to unavoidable toxins every day. Fruits, vegetables, and crops are covered in them; they are sprinkled throughout spices and seasoning; added as flavoring in beverages; and more. The various forms of toxins are damaging to your health and can impede your ability to heal from fibromyalgia. We have discussed the anti-inflammatory component of proper nutrition, but it's important to understand how and why you should detoxify your body. Proper supplementation is essential in helping you accomplish this.

Some health practitioners believe a disturbed metabolic system leads to fibromyalgia. A disturbed metabolism can present with many symptoms including fatigue, weakness, increased pain, depression, and sleep disturbances. Of course, there are many contributing factors that can interrupt metabolic function, but one major player is toxins in food.

An increase in production of internal toxins is observed in people who suffer from chronic pain. When you combine an interruption in metabolic function with toxic build up it leads to cellular dysfunction causing symptoms of pain and fatigue. Cellular cleansing and detoxification are essential to remove harmful toxins from the body.

The number of detox programs and supplement systems on the market are seemingly endless. It can be both confusing and overwhelming when deciding which one to choose. The best decision is always an educated one, so take the time to understand how they work.

It's important to choose a safe, easy, and effective detoxification system. The system we recommend is exactly that: an easy nutrition program with daily supplementation that helps detoxify your body and removes toxins safely.

The nutrition plan is simple: eat unprocessed fresh organic food made from the earth. This is easier said than done, so use this book and the online community as a guide to assist you. We have included action steps, tools, and recipes in order to make this a stress-free and successful program.

Is packaged food made from the earth? Almost all of the time, the answer is no. If you can't read, pronounce, or understand an ingredient listed on food packaging, it's likely not made from the earth. Most pre-packaged foods are filled with preservatives, additives, and chemical toxins. Choose local organic foods wherever possible. The long travel time of imported and genetically modified foods means reduced nutritional value and unknown chemical exposure.

Pesticides are also a significant source of toxins. They don't just sit on the outer surface of fruit and vegetables – they leach into the crop and can contaminate the seeds.

The Environmental Working Group (EWG) produced lists called Dirty Dozen and Clean Fifteen. These lists are handy reminders of which foods have high pesticide levels and should therefore be a guide to purchase organic, and which foods are less often contaminated by pesticides. Organic or not, washing foods with a specific soap is helpful in reducing toxicity and mold exposure. The Dirty Dozen and Clean Fifteen lists are included at the end of this chapter.

Choosing organic, non-GMO foods will lower your toxic exposure. When you follow our nutrition plan, your body's ability to remove toxins will improve naturally.

Detoxification

You can minimize your exposure to food and environmental toxins, but you can't avoid them completely. It is therefore important to detox regularly by following a detailed food plan and taking specific detox supplements, like activated charcoal, glutathione and Calcium D-Glucarate. All of these key ingredients bind to toxins and carry them out of the body rather than simply moving them to other tissues. Look for a detox supplement that has the following key ingredients.

Detox Components of Supplements

Activated Charcoal

Activated charcoal is a form of carbon that has a massive surface area along with a strong negative charge. It's been around for thousands of years and it's still used in emergency rooms today to treat acute poisoning. The use of liquid-activated charcoal in an emergency situation often results in nausea and vomiting after drinking it.

Charcoal binds to chemicals whose molecules have positive charges, including aflatoxin and other polar mycotoxins, BPA, and common pesticides. Once the chemicals attach to the charcoal, you can pass them normally. (By that, we mean poop them out!)

Charcoal can bind to the good stuff, too, so we don't recommend taking it within an hour of other supplements, especially vitamin C. Try taking charcoal pills along with a workout or sauna session. The charcoal supplement will help absorb many of the toxins you release into your GI tract.

Glutathione

If you have had fibromyalgia for some time you have probably come across glutathione, which is pronounced "gloot-a-thigh-own." Glutathione is a powerful, naturally occurring antioxidant and plays a critical role in detoxification and the immune system. Glutathione supports liver enzymes that break down mold toxins and heavy metals, protecting you from damage and toxicity.

The main reasons for declining glutathione levels are aging, environmental pollution, toxic exposure, smoking, chronic stress, poor nutrition, and some medications.

Symptoms of glutathione deficiency include but are not limited to:

- Headaches
- Brain fog

- Depression
- Dizziness
- Joint pain
- Weakness
- Lack of energy
- Frequent colds
- Sleep disturbances

Glutathione lives inside of your cells. Supplementing with glutathione is difficult because digestion destroys unfamiliar glutathione levels, but you can consume foods that enhance glutathione production and opt for a liposomal glutathione supplement that makes it through your stomach. Sulfur-rich foods like broccoli, bok choy, Brussels sprouts, and cauliflower support your body's own glutathione production. Some of the nutritional compounds that are important in producing glutathione include vitamin C, D, sulfur, and B vitamins.

Glutathione supplementation is recommended in addition to increasing glutathione food intake. Some available glutathione supplementation options are listed below.

Glutathione Supplements

Glutathione Intra-Oral Spray is absorbed through the oral mucous membrane.

Liposomal Glutathione, meaning glutathione combined with fat, is an excellent option. The

liposomes help the glutathione survive your digestive tract in order to make it to your cells.
Recommended Dosage: 200-500 mg taken 1-2 times daily, away from food.

Acetylated Glutathione is similar to liposomal glutathione in that it also survives the gut and makes it into your cells, but it has an additional advantage: it is split by cellular enzymes, so it requires no energy expenditure by your body. This form has a highly effective bioavailability.
Recommended Dosage: 200-500 mg taken 1-2 times daily, away from food.

Ultimately, the best way to determine which method works best for you is to do a blood test to determine your body's levels of glutathione before and after supplementation over a period of time.

If you have severe heavy metal or mycotoxin poisoning, talk to your healthcare practitioner about intravenous glutathione. It costs more and is less convenient than an oral supplement, but it works effectively.

Below are some of the raw foods that will help with glutathione production:

- Asparagus
- Avocado

- Spinach
- Okra
- Broccoli
- Cantaloupe
- Tomato
- Carrot
- Grapefruit
- Orange

Calcium-D Glucarate

Calcium D-Glucarate, a calcium salt found in foods, supports a crucial detoxification pathway in your liver. Small amounts are produced naturally in our body, but it can also be found in various fruits and vegetables like apples, apricots, citrus fruits, cherries, grapefruits, broccoli, Brussels sprouts, and alfalfa sprouts. Once ingested, Calcium D-Glucarate is metabolized into glucaric acid.

Glucaric acid scavenges in our body to bind to and eliminate unavoidable toxins that would otherwise wreak havoc on your health. In addition to enabling the body to rid itself of foreign elements including xenoestrogens, pollutants, and toxins, it also counteracts intestinal inflammation, helps hormone balance, and supports the immune system. Calcium-D-Glucarate is especially helpful in a detox supplement.

A Last Word on Detox Supplements

As with any supplement, you want to choose wisely. Not all detox products are created equal. While the majority help detoxify the cells, they lack binding agents to carry the toxins out of the body. Join our online community for up-to-date guidance on choosing the best product for you.

Toxicity in Your Environment

Our environment is toxic. There is no way to avoid all exposure, but you can drastically minimize it. Symptoms of fibromyalgia and other neurological illnesses are related to toxicity: levels of exposure are at an all-time high. Organs involved in our natural detox system are being overtaxed due to poor nutritional choices and as a result, most people are unable to support the proper elimination of toxins. Toxic exposure attacks the nervous system as well as the endocrine system, which manages hormone regulation and metabolism.

Medications are the number one cause of toxicity for many people in North America. North America is more medicated than ever before, and the number of people with fibromyalgia and chronic fatigue syndrome continues to increase. A healthy lifestyle is the greatest threat to pharmaceutical companies. Every drug is a chemical toxin, period. In the event that a medication is absolutely necessary, you can mitigate the damage they cause with proper nutrition and supplementation.

Personal care products contain many toxins, and some contain heavy metals. Use natural products from your local natural health store. Most health stores carry makeup and personal care product lines that are free of toxins, such as lotions, toothpaste, deodorant, feminine care products, and more.

Common household cleaning products have "caution," "warning," and "danger" labels. When using a rag to wipe the countertop, these products touch your skin and leave their chemical residue on every surface. If there are small children in your household crawling on the floors, the products you use to clean the house go onto their hands and into their mouths. Purchase only natural cleaners from your local natural health store or use the classic, age-old cleaner: vinegar.

Your yard may contain harmful contaminants. Most pesticides, insecticides, herbicides, fungicides, and fertilizers contain toxic substances. There are a variety of natural and homemade insecticide and herbicide options that can be just as effective, and much safer.

Microwaves – the convenience comes at a cost. Using a microwave to heat food decreases nutritional value. If you put plastic packaging in the microwave, chemicals can leach into the food. Heat food on the stove top if possible, and if you do use a microwave, use glass or ceramic containers.

Plastics may contain **bisphenol A** (BPA) or xenoestrogens. Xenoestrogens are synthetic or naturally occurring compounds that mimic estrogen and disrupt normal hormone levels. Xenoestrogens are found in various everyday items like makeup, the plastic containers we store our food and water in, hormones in meats and dairy, and pesticides on fruits and vegetables. Xenoestrogens are particularly detrimental to organs that are sensitive to hormones, like the uterus, breasts, and bone tissue.

Water isn't always what it appears to be! Bottled water has become popular for people on-the-go, and many believe that it's a healthier option. There is a catch. Yes, it's healthier than soda, but bottled water comes with its own set of toxic effects.

The Environmental Working Group has tested various popular bottled waters and found traces of disinfectant byproducts, industrial chemicals, prescription drugs and even bacteria. Some bottled water is simply filtered city tap water.

In many places, tap water isn't pure either. Often tap water contains chlorine, heavy metal contaminants, traces of medications such as beta-blockers, estrogen, painkillers, antidepressants and sometimes even lead.

Digestive issues such as nausea, diarrhea, constipation, abdominal pain, bloating, and gas are often conditions that coexist with fibromyalgia. Chlorine is added to tap water to kill bacteria in the water. When you drink chlorinated water, it destroys both the good and bad bacteria in your body and disrupts your natural intestinal flora balance. Removing chlorine from your drinking water with a filter and adding in a probiotic supplement is a good start to restore digestive homeostasis.

In addition to the various substances found in bottled water, consider the health effects of the plastic bottles themselves. Single-serve containers made of polyethylene terephthalate known as PET plastic (labeled #1 on the bottom of the container) leach additional contaminants into the water. One study investigated the claim that plastics used for water bottles leach antimony. Antimony is a regulated contaminant that can have both acute and chronic health effects like depression, dizziness, and nausea. Their findings showed that there is a small release of antimony from the plastic bottle into the water. However, the majority of the release takes place when the water bottle is exposed to high temperatures. For example, summertime temperatures inside of vehicles and storage areas.

Solution

- Know your city water source by reviewing city testing. Periodically test the water in your home.
- Choose a good quality filter for your tap. There are many choices when it comes to low-cost carbon filters, but you get what you pay for. Research before buying. Keep in mind, something is better than nothing. The most effective water filter system you can choose is reverse osmosis. You can have a reverse osmosis system installed on a specific tap in your home or have a large home system installed that filters all water coming into the home. Alternatively, an economical option that is a bit more labor intensive is to visit a reverse osmosis depot in your town and have glass or BPA-free water jugs filled. You can use a pump or water cooler for conveniently dispensing the drinking water.
- Choose to store filtered water in a glass or BPA free container when cooling in the fridge or on the go during the day.

Heavy Metal Exposures

Are You Toxic?

To determine if you are at risk and require a heavy metals detox, ask yourself these questions:

- Do you cook with aluminum cookware?
- Do you have, or have you had mercury fillings in your teeth?
- Do you, or have you lived in a house with old galvanized water pipes? Or do you drink from drinking fountains in older buildings?
- Are you a smoker or are you exposed to secondhand smoke?
- Have you ever worked in a factory around toxic metals, or welded?
- Do you have a hobby that uses lead or solder, such as creating stained glass windows, or ceramics?
- Have you renovated an old house? Scraped or removed old paint?
- Do you live or work on a farm, or did you grow up on a farm?
- Have you had any surgical metal implants?

Toxic metals undermine the immune system and cause many physical, mental, emotional, and behavioral symptoms. Metal allergies are common in fibromyalgia patients, and the most common sensitivities are to nickel, inorganic mercury, cadmium, and lead. Heavy metals result in inflammation, which is common in those with fibromyalgia. Heavy metals are attackers and their targets are the central nervous system; exposure produces oxidative stress which results in neurological changes in the brain. The World Health Organization states that heavy metals have "effects on the nervous, digestive, and immune systems." Reduced metal exposure results in improved health.

Exposure to toxic heavy metals occurs through air, food, and water. Take a closer look at the list below and think about how you may be exposed.

Cadmium exposure is mostly from cigarette smoking, and small amounts can come from eating certain foods grown in contaminated soil.

Aluminum exposure can be through consumption of compounds that are added during processing of foods, such as flour, baking powder, coloring agents, anti-caking agents, and drinking water.
Aluminum is also found in some cosmetics, antiperspirants, and pharmaceuticals such as antacids, buffered aspirin, and vaccines. Soda cans, aluminum foil, and cookware such as Teflon pans often contain aluminum. Exposure is often high in those who work and live in a mining environment, work in factories, or are welders.

Mercury is a heavy metal and most people are aware of its dangers. The majority of controllable mercury exposure is in the form of dental amalgam fillings and coal-burning power plants. It is recommended that pregnant women, nursing mothers, and young children avoid certain types of fish because of the mercury content. High mercury fish includes tuna, shark, swordfish, king mackerel, and tilefish.

Fish low in mercury include shrimp, salmon, pollock, catfish, anchovies, and sardines. The general rule for fish is to minimize consumption of large predatory fish and stick to the smaller fish.

Mercury is also found in batteries, old thermometers, barometers, electric switches, and compact fluorescent light bulbs. If a mercury light bulb breaks, take caution. First, remove people and pets from the room. Leave the room for fifteen minutes and turn off central air for several hours. Being careful to not touch bulb material with bare hands, place the broken pieces in a glass jar with a metal lid and check with your local government on disposal requirements.

Antimony is often found in industrial emissions and coal-burning cities. Antimony is often partnered with lead in the production of products and used in batteries, metals, flame-proofing materials, paints, ceramic enamels, glass, and pottery.

Lead exposure can occur through occupational and environmental sources generated by burning lead-containing materials. For example, during smelting, recycling, stripping leaded paint, and using leaded gasoline. More common exposure is through ingestion of lead-contaminated dust, water from old leaded pipes, and food from lead- glazed or lead-soldered containers. Lead can also be found in some cosmetics and medicines.

Take your shoes off in the home to avoid lead-contaminated soil from being tracked through the house. If you have old lead pipes in your home, run them with cold water in the morning for a few minutes before using the water, or better yet – use a water filter! Daily intake or supplementation of calcium, vitamin C, and iron will help keep lead from being absorbed.

Arsenic has also been found in well-water, industrial processes, and tobacco smoke. Eighty percent of dietary arsenic intake is through meat, fish, and poultry.

Heavy Metal Testing

There are three ways to test for heavy metals—hair analysis, blood, and urine testing. Each test provides valuable but different information. Hair analysis looks at chronic toxic exposure. Blood analysis assesses acute exposure. Urine analysis provides a measurement of the body's ability to eliminate heavy metals and environmental toxins. Hair and urine analysis will be of most value for those suffering from chronic symptoms. These tests can be performed or ordered by an appropriate healthcare practitioner. For some, heavy metal testing will come back negative, showing that heavy metals are not a contributing culprit to your situation, however, others may be surprised to learn of toxicity that may be aggravating their nervous system. It's worth testing for.

Pesticides

Pesticides are used to control pests by poisoning them. Some pesticides are poisonous and toxic to humans as well. Picture the farm workers wearing full-body hazmat suits as they spray crops and consider the safety of ingesting those pesticides when you eat fruits and vegetables. If someone wore a hazmat suit when handling it, you probably don't want to eat it. Pesticides persist on some foods more than others, even after they are washed and peeled. We again refer to the Dirty Dozen and Clean Fifteen list.

EWG'S 2020
DIRTY 12™

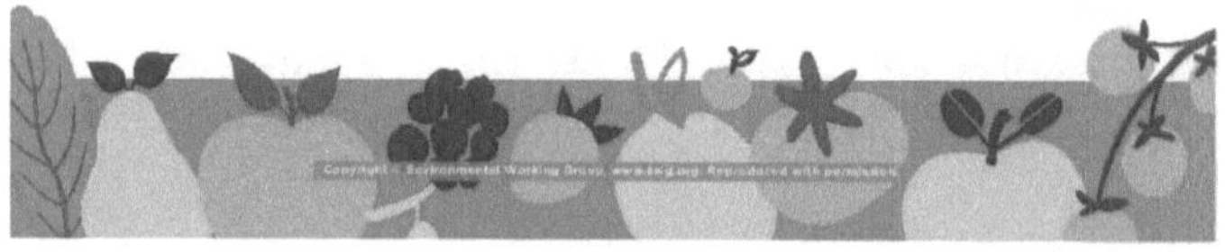

1. Strawberries
2. Spinach
3. Kale
4. Nectarines
5. Apples
6. Grapes
7. Peaches
8. Cherries
9. Pears
10. Tomatoes
11. Celery
12. Potatoes

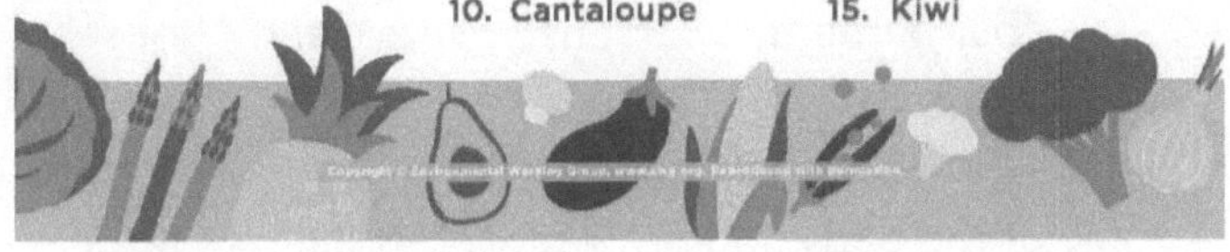

Visit https://www.ewg.org/ for the most current updates.

What to Do

It's impossible to entirely avoid exposure to toxins, but it's worth taking the steps to minimize and mitigate exposure. Here are some action steps to take:

- Undergo heavy metal testing with blood, urine and hair samples
- Drink only filtered water
- Minimize your exposure to toxins in your environment, personal care, and household products
- Take a detoxifying supplement to pull toxins out of the body and protect against daily exposures
- Consume organic and natural foods that don't add to the toxic load
- Use an infrared sauna

THE NERVOUS SYSTEM

The nervous system consists of the brain, spinal cord, and nerves. It controls every cell, gland, organ, and tissue in the body. It is your master system, controlling all of the body's function and healing.

The nervous system is like a highway along which the brain is constantly sending and receiving information to and from the body. The brain learns what the body needs through the nervous system, and then responds appropriately to fulfill those needs.

The nervous system is divided into two parts: the central, and the peripheral. The central nervous system is made up of the brain, brainstem, and spinal cord, while the peripheral nervous system consists of the nerves I your body. When this two-way communication highway between your brain and body is free of interference, your body is able to function smoothly and heal optimally.

Think of a light on a dimmer switch. When you dim the switch, you are interfering with the transmission of electrical energy to the light bulb. When the light switch is turned on full you give the bulb 100% light potential. Apply this metaphor to your nervous system. If there is interference to the transmission of nerve energy, the body cannot function optimally.

The brain and spinal cord are protected by the skull, the spine, and the spinal column. The spine is made up of twenty-four vertebrae, which are small, mobile bones. We are exposed to physical, emotional, and chemical stress on a daily basis. This stress can create hyperactivity of the nerve roots along the spine which in turn creates muscle tension. Tight muscles have the strength to move bones, and this tightness can move the vertebrae slightly out of alignment. When a vertebra is out of alignment its range of motion is limited, and there is additional stress and tension to the spinal cord and surrounding nerves.

Autonomic Nervous System

The autonomic nervous system provides nerve supply to our smooth muscles and glands, controlling the function of our internal organs. This control system functions unconsciously and reflexively, constantly working to regulate critical body processes behind the scenes.

YELLOW = SYMPATHETIC / GREEN = PARASYMPATHETIC

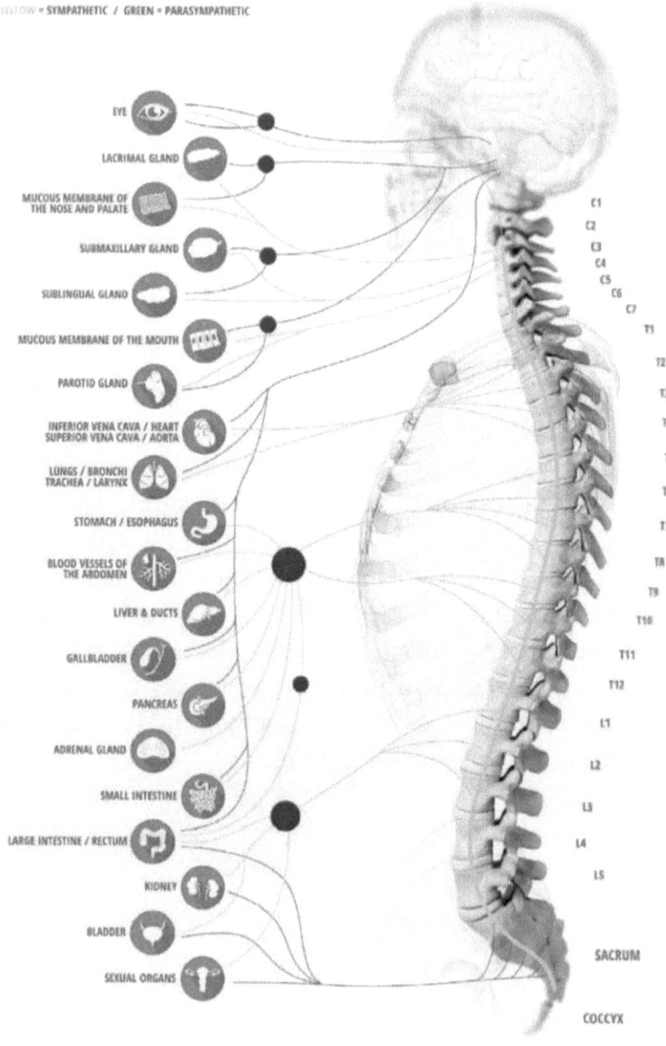

When the vertebrae are misaligned and restricted, it creates "traffic congestion" on the two-way highway of communication between your brain and your body. Over time, this creates more damage to the spine, puts pressure on the nervous system, and decreases health of cells, organs, and tissues. When this happens, it is harder for the body to produce healthy cells and detoxify, which is critical for patients with fibromyalgia.

Symptoms like headaches, pain, digestive issues, and immune system problems are commonly due to nerve pressure caused by spinal misalignment. It is vital to maintain a nervous system free of stress and interference by taking care of what protects your nervous system: your spine. Your body is resilient – it doesn't want you to be in pain. If you leave the problem long enough, your body will give you the symptoms to let you know.

Just as proper dental hygiene is important the moment you start having teeth, the best time to start caring for the spine and nervous system is during your formative years. Countless patients have arrived at our clinic after years of damage and say "I wish someone had told me this thirty years ago!"

Doctors of Chiropractic (or Doctors of Cause) focus on the root cause of health disorders. The primary objective with chiropractic care is to correct any misalignments to your spinal column, correct the underlying cause of stress to your nervous system, and remove interference to your body to restore normal function. This allows the body to begin its own natural healing process.

Chiropractors use specific techniques, or adjustments, to restore proper spinal mechanics and free up the nervous system. Just like proper nutrition and exercise, chiropractic is not just a treatment but a lifestyle. Even if a chiropractor alleviates your symptoms, it's important that you continue to take care of your body.

Your First Visit

After a comprehensive consultation and getting to know your personal history, your chiropractor will examine you with a system of analysis to determine if there are areas of spinal misalignment causing nerve interference. The most common forms of analysis chiropractors use are:

1) X Rays
2) Postural evaluation
3) EMG (electromyography)
4) Thermography
5) Range of motion
6) Muscle tests

Based on this analysis, your chiropractor will identify the underlying cause of your problem and know where to apply specific adjustments in order to restore proper alignment.

Proper alignment will minimize spinal decay and degeneration, allowing the discs to maintain proper hydration.

Chronic pain can place an incredible amount of stress on your body, and this can manifest into other conditions. That's why we frequently see fibromyalgia patients who also experience a complex range of other health issues. Rather than masking and patching up these health issues with medications, your chiropractor will uncover and correct the cause. Over-the-counter medications for pain such as acetaminophen and ibuprofen are chemical stressors and toxins that increase cardiovascular risk and kidney problems. Fibromyalgia patients most commonly turn to prescription drugs like Lyrica, Cymbalta, and Savella, which also increase your risk of cardiovascular disease in addition to digestive problems, insomnia, and even suicidal thoughts.

Regular chiropractic care also lowers inflammation in the body, which is great news for those suffering from symptoms.

The nervous system plays a role in immune system function. A healthy nervous system will allow the body to better fight off the bacteria and viruses commonly seen among fibromyalgia patients.

Therefore, it is important to ensure the best possible function of your nervous system.

Chiropractic: The Facts

    a. Improves lung function
    b. Improves autonomic tone
    c. Decreases blood markers of inflammation
    d. Decreases chest pain

Many patients see a chiropractor for the first time after their body has accumulated years of damage. These chronic conditions require time to correct the underlying cause and allow your body to heal, so be patient and stick with your treatments.

Chiropractic is one of the safest practices in health care. Studies have repeatedly demonstrated the efficacy and safety of chiropractic for conditions related to the spine. The safety of chiropractic is underpinned by the fact that chiropractors pay a mere fraction in malpractice insurance when compared to their medical counterparts.

Spinal Health Questionnaire

Check off any of the following that apply to you.

- o Have you given birth? Did you have a challenging birth process? (Including the use of medical intervention such as the use of forceps, suction, C-section, etc.)
- o Have you ever suffered from a sporting injury?
- o Have you ever had a concussion?
- o Have you ever been in a vehicle collision or other impact trauma?
- o Do you have poor posture while sitting or standing?
- o Do you drive or sit at a computer for more than three hours a day?
- o Do you experience high levels of physical, chemical, or emotional stress?
- o Do you sleep on your stomach?
- o Do you experience tight, stiff, or weak muscles?

If you checked off any of the above, it's time to get a spinal evaluation! Misalignments or dysfunction of spinal joints are common.

Take action. Go to the "find a practitioner" at familyhealthadvocacy.com.

Sharon's Story

I'm a 35-year-old mother of two. I had a number of symptoms, the worst of which were migraines that would completely incapacitate me. I would spend hours in my room with all of the lights off. Many days were ruined. I was always feeling stiff and in pain. I would usually rely on medications, but they never really worked.

Now after getting my spine in alignment and removing nervous system stress, as well as following Dr. Casey and Dr. Morgan's recommendations, I no longer use medications. I don't get migraines anymore or experience any of the stiffness and pain. I have experienced a complete 180 with my health. Most of all, I appreciate all of the time and education I received from the doctors.

Postural / Physical Stress

It's easy to understand how physical trauma such as a car accident, fall, or sporting injury can cause structural and functional damage to your body resulting in acute or chronic pain. However, the repetitive strain from poor posture is often overlooked as something that could be causing everyday pain. Some may experience pain creep up the moment they sit down at a computer or use their phone. Others may not experience any negative effects from poor posture even after sitting for a full eight-hour workday. Either way, over time, the stress of poor posture causes changes to your spine.

Poor posture often results in neck, mid-back, and lower back pain, as well as hip pain, headaches, and numbness or tingling in your arms and legs. Chronic postural issues can cause "upper crossed syndrome," which is often referred to as "student or corporate syndrome."

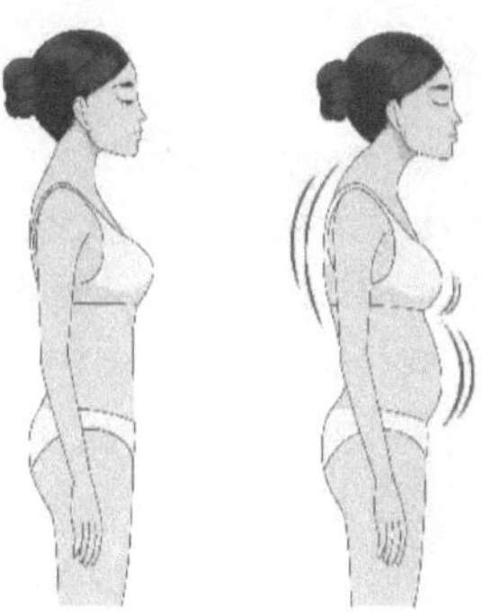

As healthcare practitioners, we are constantly moving around the office throughout our day. It's rare to find us sitting for periods longer than one hour. Writing this book has required prolonged sitting, which has been a significant change in our daily posture. This reminded us of how delicate our bodies are, and how consistent sedentary postures result in pain. We took many breaks to stretch, use our acu-balls, and foam roll. We increased our chiropractic care and received additional therapies as well.

It's not uncommon for people to spend forty hours a week at work on a computer station, plus time on their personal devices such as phones, tablets, and laptops. For most people that results in over fifty hours a week on a technological device, and that's not even including driving or television time. Add another fifty hours a week in bed in a poor sleep position and it's easy to see how a hundred or more hours a week of poor posture can negate the few hours you have dedicated to taking care of yourself with stretching and exercise.

It's important to stay conscious of your posture throughout the day. Reducing postural stresses will maximize the benefits of self-care and therapy. The result? An accumulation of positive change.

Optimizing Your Workstation

Chair

Choose a chair that supports the natural curvatures of your spine. If possible, choose one made with a breathable fabric. The most important thing is to use a chair with low back support. The lower back is slightly curved inward, like a C, so our chairs shouldn't be straight or without support. If you do not have lumbar support in your chair, try sitting on an inflatable cushion, or place a rolled-up hand towel or small pillow against your low back. This lumbar support will prevent slouching, taking pressure off of your low back and neck.

Adjust the seat height so your feet are flat on the floor or on a footrest to ensure the knees are parallel to the hips. If you find your feet are dangling, lower the seat or use a footrest. If a footrest is not available, try using a stack of books or a box instead. Adjust the armrests so that your shoulders are relaxed. Ideally, your elbows will be bent 90-100 degrees. When you sit in the chair, push your hips as far back as they can go.

Mouse and Keyboard

It's important that all frequently used items such as keyboard, mouse, and telephone are close to your body in order to minimize reaching. When you reach and extend your elbows beyond 100 degrees, you put tension and stress on the neck and upper back. Bring your chair closer to the desk and keyboard or install a keyboard tray and pull it out closer to you as you sit. If you need to use a less frequently used item like the printer, stand up and move closer to the item to minimize reaching.

Place your keyboard and mouse close to one another and on the same surface. Use a wrist pad or palm support to ensure your wrists stay in a neutral position. While typing, keep your elbows bent 90-100 degrees, your arms close to your body, and your wrists in a neutral position at or below elbow level.

Feeling ambidextrous? Try alternating the mouse pad and phone to either side of the keyboard periodically.

Computer Monitor and Telephone

The position of your monitor has a huge impact on your posture. Center the monitor directly in front of you, approximately one arm's length away. The top of the monitor should be two-three inches above seated eye level. Avoid any rotation in the neck or body while sitting at your desk looking at your monitor.

Be mindful of your monitor position with regards to sunlight, interior lighting, and glare. If your resources allow, use a glass glare or light filter for the screen. Place your monitor so that bright light is to the side.

On the phone a lot? Invest in a headset or use speakerphone if your space allows for it. Avoid cradling the phone between your head and neck or shoulder.

Laptop

Ideally, you are using a desktop that provides more efficient ergonomic set-up. However, depending on location demands, you may be limited to a laptop. If this is you, invest in modifications to use with the laptop in your main office space.

    i.   Raise the height of the laptop by setting it on a riser, footstool, or stack of books
   ii.   Use an external keyboard and mouse

And... Break!

Get up and move around for at least five minutes every half hour or so. Sometimes just walking to a water station, standing while you are on the phone or stepping aside to stretch will make the difference, resulting in a pain-free and productive day.

Justin's Story

I'm 23 years old and have been working in a grocery store for the past few years. I was really struggling on the job. My job required a lot of bending and lifting, which I found extremely difficult as I was in so much pain. I was experiencing pain all over my body, but it was mostly in my back. The pain was so bad it caused me to walk with a slant and lean to one side. It was terrible and embarrassing.

Ever since I started following the protocol, work has gotten so much better. I haven't missed a day of work and am rarely, if ever, in pain. I am now more conscious about how to bend and lift properly so that I can continue to experience the benefits of Dr. Casey and Morgan's advice. I'm now able to walk normally and with confidence. I have a lot more energy to be active, exercise, and play sports. I would recommend this program to anyone that is suffering similarly to the way I was. It has changed my life!

Optimizing Ergonomics of Cell Phone Use

The "smartphone slump" has become an epidemic among cell phone users, and so has the pain and health problems associated with it. Teenagers and children are coming into our clinic complaining of neck and back pain along with headaches. It's incredible watching these young people as they sit in our waiting room, slouched over their phones. They aren't even aware that they're here to fix a problem they're actively perpetuating. It has been said that sitting is the new smoking, however it's not sitting in itself but the poor posture that often goes along with it that is damaging.

Chief of Spine Surgery at New York Spine Surgery and Rehabilitation Medicine, Dr. Kenneth Hansraj, has found that as you flex your head forward out of the natural curve, the weight on the spine dramatically increases. Imagine standing up and holding a bowling ball against your chest. Heavy, but doable. Now imagine holding the bowling ball in front of you with your arms stretched out. Starting to shake?

The average human head weighs around 10lbs, pretty close to the weight of a bowling ball. As your head shifts further forward and away from your body, the heavier the weight on your spine and stress on the nervous system. These added stresses lead to early wear and tear, degeneration, and the associated symptoms of neck and back pain, headaches, numbness and tingling, weakness into the arms, chest tightness, dizziness and so on.

This diagram shows the relationship between cell phone posture and tension on the spine based on Dr. Hansraj's research.

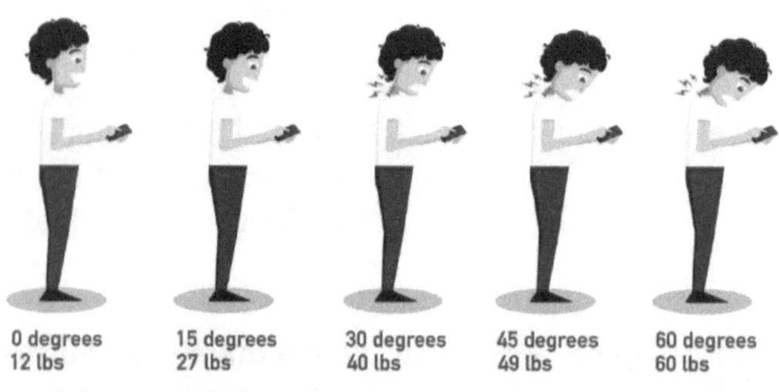

It is impossible in our world to avoid cell phone use. However, postural corrections and reduction in hours spent on devices should be made.

Here are some life-changing tips:

1. Hold your phone up at eye level. If you have shoulder pain, you may find it easier to hold the phone just below eye level, but be sure to have your eyes gaze downwards rather than shifting your head and neck towards the phone.
2. Surfing the internet and checking emails while at home? Use your computer!

3. Surfing the internet on your phone? Lay down on your back with your knees bent and feet on the floor. Hold your phone over your face. This position allows your neck and shoulders to be straight and relaxed on the floor. Be sure not to make the mistake we have and hold onto your phone securely!

4. My personal favorite: use voice to text when messaging!

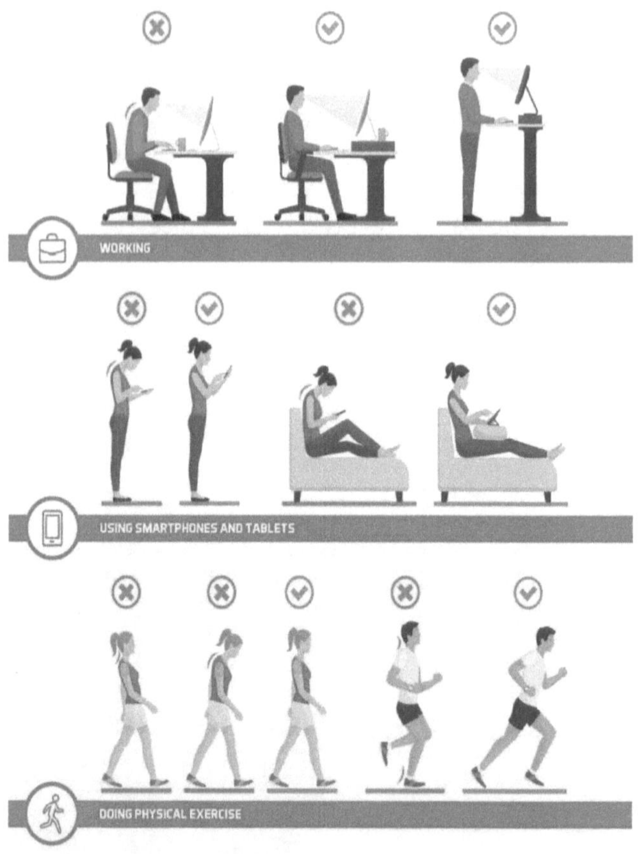

How is your posture? Be mindful of your body position throughout your day, at work, while exercising, and while using technology at home. This will reduce strain and pain.

Optimizing Your Sleep Time

Too much or too little sleep has been linked to an array of health problems. Most people lay in bed for an average of seven hours a night, whether they are sleeping or counting sheep. Your sleep position can affect your quality of sleep, and either contribute to or alleviate pain. When you are going to sleep, be mindful of proper spinal alignment. Ask yourself if you were standing for six to seven hours in this position, would you develop aches and pains?

First of all, stomach sleeping is a big no-no. When you lay on your stomach, your head is rotated for hours, jamming the spinal joints and irritating the connected nerves. Sleeping in this position also hyperextends the natural curve in your lower back which further compresses the joints.

Sleeping on your back with neck, low back and knee support is the ideal sleep position for the spine. A common mistake is using too many pillows, or supports that are too large or soft. However, for the population that snores or has sleep apnea, back sleeping may prove difficult.

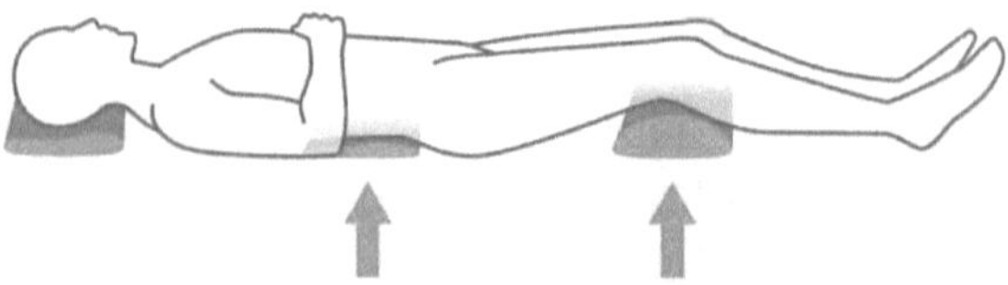

While back sleeping is preferred, side sleeping is definitely allowed! This is the most common sleep position. Proper pillow choice is key to side sleeping: when the pillow is too thin, we tend to raise an arm to rest the head. This restricts blood flow to the arm and irritates nerves in the neck, which can cause pain and numbness. If you sleep on your side, try placing a pillow between your knees to take stress off your pelvic area and lower back. If you experience upper back or shoulder discomfort, place a pillow in front of your chest and rest your arm on it.

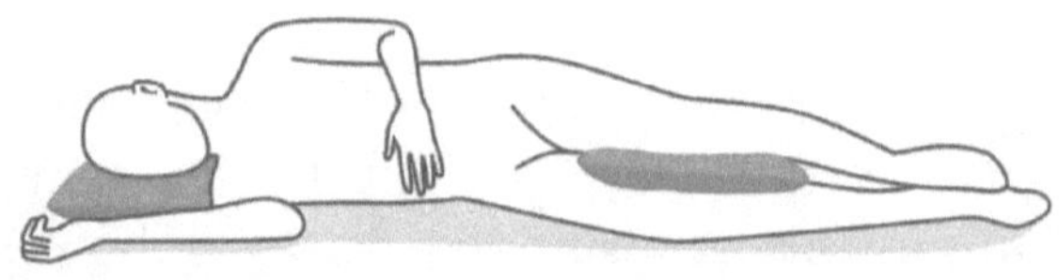

Pillow Talk: Optimizing Ergonomics of Sleep Posture

The cervical 'C' curve in your neck is small and doesn't need much support in order to be in a healthy, stable position. When sleeping on your back, try rolling up a hand towel or a thin pillow into the curve. For side sleepers, proper pillow use is recommended. Choosing the right pillow is difficult: the tricky part is that there's no perfect pillow for everyone, because everybody has a different shoulder to neck measurement ratio. We encourage patients to use the pillow test.

Pillow test: Stand with one shoulder against the wall. Place the pillow between the wall and your neck. Completely relax your neck and shoulders allowing your head to fall gently into the pillow against the wall. Do not push your head into the pillow, simply let gravity take its course. Your head should not be tilted, and there should only be a lateral shift in your neck of two to three inches. If there is a larger shift, the spine is being stressed and this isn't the pillow for you. If you find that there is no lateral movement of your head, the pillow is too thick and can cause awkward postural stress on the spine as well.

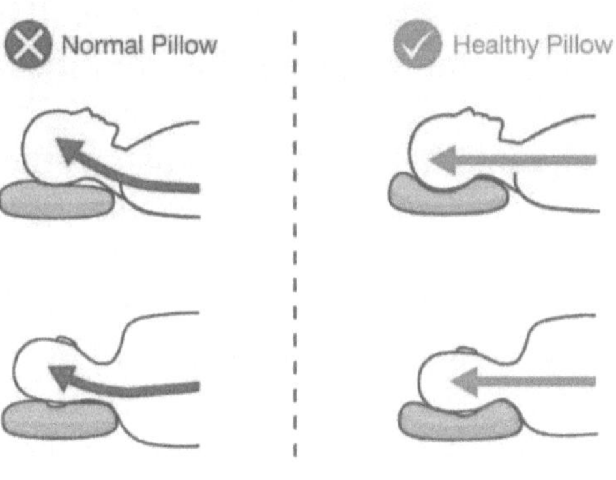

Deep Sleep!

Deep sleep is essential for healing. Sleep disturbances and chronic fatigue are among the most common symptoms of fibromyalgia. Those suffering from fibromyalgia are often caught in a difficult loop: pain affects quality sleep, and sleep deprivation exacerbates pain. This is a cycle that needs to be broken. In one study, a group of people were deprived of sleep for three consecutive days. Participants reported:

> "...decreased pain threshold, increased discomfort, fatigue, and an inflammatory flare response in the skin. These results suggest that disrupted sleep is probably an important factor in the pathophysiology of symptoms in fibromyalgia."

Proper sleep is crucial for proper organ function, clear thinking, motor function, hormone regulation, metabolism, increased energy, and overall health – all of which are common symptoms of fibromyalgia.

The body's internal clock is known as the circadian rhythm, and it cycles between sleepiness and alertness according to hormone messengers, cortisol and melatonin, sent by the brain. Cortisol and serotonin are released mostly in the early part of the day to help with alertness, while melatonin is released at the end of the day to help with sleep.

These hormones also affect blood pressure, muscle strength, alertness, reaction time, bowel movements, sleep rhythm, and body temperature.

If you experience difficulty sleeping, here are a few tips to improve your quality of sleep.

- *Establish a routine.* Aim to have a bedtime and wake up time that is consistent daily. Ideally, work with the sun's rhythm. Try to be in bed by 10 p.m. On your days off, avoid sleeping in as this will disrupt your routine. If you are a napper, be smart about it. Limit your naps to 15-20 minutes to avoid going into a deep sleep and affecting your energy levels and routine for the rest of the day.
- *Make your room as dark as possible.* Use heavy curtains, turn off the nightlight, sleep with a mask, and turn off electronics. Your brain releases melatonin when it's dark. Melatonin is responsible for making you feel sleepy. When there is too much light, the brain doesn't release as much melatonin, which affects your sleep-wake cycle and makes you feel more alert.
- *Take melatonin and magnesium supplements.* These will help improve relaxation and enhance sleep quality. See the Nutrition section for dosing recommendations and additional benefits.
- *Use lavender as a supplement or essential oil.* Lavender is well known for having an ability to induce a calming and relaxing effect to improve

sleep. Try taking a bath with some lavender essential oil or put a few drops of the oil near your pillow.

- *Drink warm beverages.* Enjoy a mug of calming herbal caffeine-free tea or hot lemon water.
- *Avoid screen time.* Put away your cell phone and computer and avoid TV within 1-2 hours of bedtime. If you need to use your cell phone, choose to use the "night-time" light altering mode.
- *Establish a bedtime ritual.* Listen to relaxing music, read, take a warm Epsom salt bath, do some gentle stretches, meditate, and of course complete your gratitude list in your journal.
- *Shortly after waking up, expose yourself to bright sunlight.* Take the dog for a walk, have breakfast by a sunlit window or have coffee outside. This will help your brain stay in the rhythm of the sleep-wake cycle and result in you being more alert during the day.
- *Exercise.* Keep strenuous activity to the daytime or in a well-lit area at night.
- *Avoid caffeine.* Caffeinated drinks can cause sleep problems up to ten hours after consumption. Avoid alcohol as well. It may help you fall asleep but will interfere with your sleep cycle.
- *Maintain a proper sleep posture,* as discussed in this chapter.
- *Work on muscle relaxation with deep breathing.* If you're in bed and find yourself counting sheep instead of sleeping, try a full-body meditation.

Start with your toes and slowly work your way up to your head. Tense all the muscles in each part of your body as tightly as you can as you breathe in slowly, then completely relax as you exhale slowly. Visualize your muscles releasing all tension and peacefully falling to sleep as you relax them.

Farah's Story

I'm 43 years old and a mother of four. I've been working as a pharmacist for ten years now. I never felt anyone understood what I was going through when I was experiencing my symptoms. I had a lot of pain in my wrists, feet, and back. I was always tired with very little energy. My sleep was terrible, and every single day was a challenge to get through. I had been to a number of doctors and was prescribed Lyrica but had to stop taking it because I started experiencing a lot of dizziness. I had to find another solution to my problem. I followed Dr. Casey and Dr. Morgan's recommendations and it changed everything for me. Physically, I am able to sit in a chair properly which I wasn't able to do before due to pain. I can stand and walk for long periods as well as reach my arms above my head without any pain. I am sleeping so much better and through the night which has resulted in a huge boost in energy and strength throughout the day. My mood is a lot better and I have had a huge reduction in stress. I am now able to enjoy the little things in life and living as I was meant to!

EXERCISE

We know that exercise and being active is good for us, but when struggling with painful symptoms of fibromyalgia you may avoid exercise altogether. That's totally understandable, but we want to help you find some gentle ways to ease yourself back into physical activity. Exercise has been shown to relieve the suffering of fibromyalgia, and it's time to work towards a more active lifestyle doing the things you love.

The fear of exercise typically comes from past experience. In addition to the fear of more pain, many people simply struggle with the energy to just show up and do it. The mental blocks making it difficult to incorporate exercise into your daily routine are very real and can be even more of an obstacle than the physical block. If this resonates with you, flip back to the chapter on mindset, work on those exercises, and tackle the mental block keeping you from exercising.

The simplest advice we can give you is this: just show up. You may be telling yourself every excuse in the book (not this book!) on why you can't exercise today. "I don't have time, it's raining, I'm in too much pain, I don't want to hurt more tomorrow," etc. Regardless of what negative belief system you've fallen into, just show up. If your goal is to go for a walk, get your running shoes on and step outside. If you have a yoga mat in the spare room, put on some leggings and go into that room. If it's the gym, pack your bag, drive to the gym, and go inside. If it's the tennis court, get your racket and balls and show up to the court. Once you are there, at the place you intend to exercise, *then* decide if you are going to be active and exercise.

We have never shown up and not done anything, and we also can't remember a time that we chose to be active and regretted it. So at least show up: that's the first and most important step.

The benefits of exercise for those suffering from fibromyalgia are countless. In one study, mild aerobic exercise was found to have an effect on rewiring the nervous system and how it interprets stimuli like touch, which provided relief from chronic pain. Exercise also improves memory and mental clarity.

When dealing with chronic pain, moving your body may be something you want to avoid altogether. It's not going to be easy at first, but with commitment and staying consistent you will find it gets easier and you will feel better with time.

Some of our patients had never exercised before, and we have helped them perform simple exercises and activities and experience incredible results with their quality of life. Over time, we helped them slowly increase the difficulty and length of their daily activities. With a sedentary lifestyle, we become less mobile, less flexible, and more stiff and rigid until finally rigor mortis sets in. Which means you're dead! Movement is literally life, so get moving!

Dr. Daniel Clauw, professor of anesthesiology and medicine at the University of Michigan, stated: "Exercise is one of the most effective treatments for fibromyalgia." We know that not exercising can worsen chronic pain syndromes, but too much too soon can do the same. Start light, and focus on stretching, strengthening, mobility, and improved posture.

Benefits of Exercise

Exercise is necessary for re-training your nervous system. As discussed previously in this book, physical, chemical, and emotional stresses have an accumulative effect on your body and interfere with your nervous system, affecting the way it perceives stimuli. Now it's time to re-educate your brain and make you the best version of yourself again.

Keeping in motion also:

- Maintains and improves bone mass
- Releases serotonin and endorphins
- Improves balance
- Reduces stress
- Increases strength
- Reduces cortisol levels, therefore reducing inflammation
- Reduces pain
- Improves sleep
- Controls your weight, which is important to reducing the pain of fibromyalgia
- Rewires your brain and its perception of pain
- Boosts glutathione levels

Mary's Story

I have lived the typical fibromyalgia story. I spent over a decade severely exhausted and weak. Exhaustion kept me from doing any form of exercise or having any social life. I used to take two or three long naps every day. I suffered from insomnia at night and tried everything naturally and medically to get myself into a normal sleep schedule. My memory was embarrassing. I felt like I had a cloud wrapped around my brain and I could not think straight.

My medical doctor said that nothing was physically wrong with me and diagnosed me with depression. I didn't feel sad or depressed. I felt exhausted and frustrated, but not sad. I felt like no one else could understand me, never mind figure out what was causing this. After getting no relief from the medications, two years later I was diagnosed with fibromyalgia.

My mom was seeing Dr. Morgan and Dr. Casey and asked them to call me to provide some advice. They did. I felt like going into their office was worth the time because I felt like someone was going to listen. I saw the doctors in the office and after extensive testing, they introduced me to an easy-to-

follow program. I did not expect the results that I received. After a month of care, I finally had my first full six hours of sleep through the night. Within two months I had cut my naps down to one 15-minute power nap. I felt like I could remember conversations I was having and following through with the things I said I would do.

Now, after six months of care, I got a part-time job and have joined the gym. I have routine back in my life. The structure has helped build my self-worth. I have reconnected with my two best friends and have the energy to spend time with them on a weekly basis.

Where to Start

Here are some places you might begin your exercise journey.

Walk with swagger!

To walk with swagger is to walk with pride, confidence, and certainty. Have confidence and pride in the health you are working towards and acknowledge these steps in your daily milestones. We recommend most of our fibromyalgia patients start their personal exercise program with walking. It's a feasible activity since it's something most people do every day, to some degree – we're just encouraging you to do more of it!

Walking is a low impact activity, so it doesn't create major stress on your joints. It's a form of aerobic activity, gets oxygen to your muscles, and relieves pain. Walking will help strengthen your bones and muscles and increase your proprioception (balance and coordination). And as with any exercise, it can also improve your mood.

We recommend starting with short walks of approximately ten minutes a day, then slowly increase the time until you're walking thirty minutes a day.

Get wet!

Not all fibromyalgia sufferers can dive headfirst into a workout program at the gym... so make it a pool!

Exercising in the pool is easier on the body and can provide even more relief from fibromyalgia symptoms than performing the same exercises outside of the water. This is because water creates a buoyancy which decreases the amount of stress on the joints while increasing strength, flexibility, general mobility, and circulation.

A bit of a stretch!

People tend to think of stretching as something you only do before and after exercising, but really, it's something that should be done daily regardless of any other workout. Stretching increases circulation, re-energizes the body, and improves coordination and mobility while decreasing the symptoms of pain.

Lift off!

Some of our fibromyalgia patients are surprised when we tell them that strength training with weights can relieve fibromyalgia pain. Weights, machines, resistance bands, or any form of strength training have huge health benefits when done properly. We recommend starting light with two-pound weights and slowly increasing the weight as you get stronger. Not only will your muscles strengthen but so will your bones. Strength training can help improve posture, sleep, mood, and overall energy. It can also reduce inflammation, which is key for fibromyalgia sufferers.

Yoga and Meditation

Yoga is the practice of adopting specific body postures in combination with breathing exercises in order to achieve health and relaxation. Meditation is a component of yoga, with a focus on mental relaxation and concentration. The practice gives a lot of attention to your thoughts and breathing. Yoga and meditation have been shown to improve symptoms of pain and fatigue in fibromyalgia sufferers, and more specifically, symptoms of stiffness, anxiety, and depression. Remember, positive thoughts help you get well and stay well.

Tai Chi

Tai chi is based on ancient principles of integrating the mind with the body, with a focus on controlling movements and breathing. Tai chi nurtures the life energy in the body known as "qi." The practice of tai chi has demonstrated significant improvements in pain, tenderness, fatigue, and overall quality of life in individuals with fibromyalgia. The practice is also very gentle and low impact, making it tolerable for those suffering from fibromyalgia.

Therapeutic Mobility Exercises and Stretches

Mobility exercises and stretching help combat unavoidable physical stress everyone experiences. The following exercises are designed for the larger muscle groups that commonly endure postural stress from prolonged periods of sitting and standing. Holding these positions for around thirty seconds each will also provide relief of emotional stress and tension. While holding the stretch, focus on taking deep breaths and relaxing your muscles. Always stretch both sides.

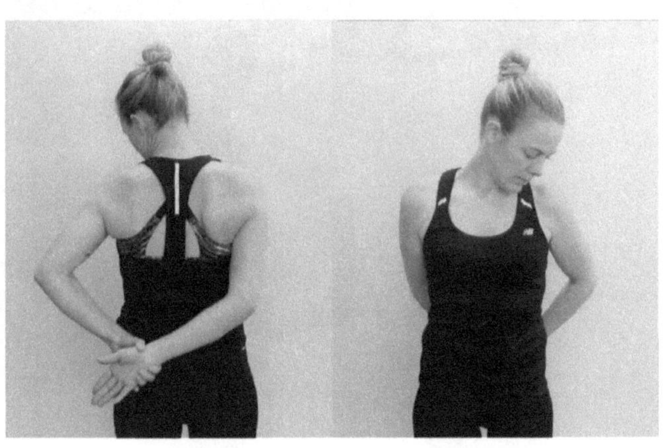

Exercise 1 Back view   Exercise 1 Front view

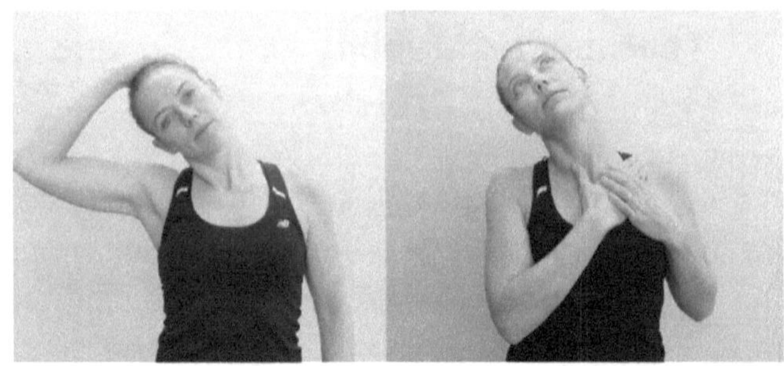

Exercise 2   Exercise 3

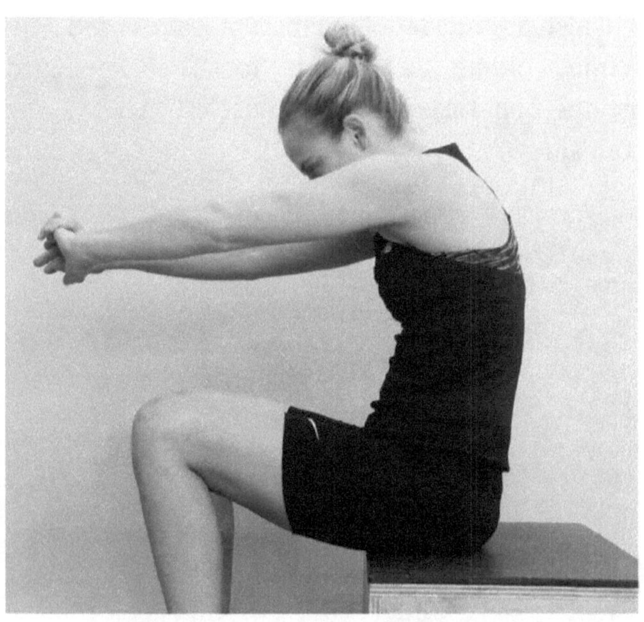

Exercise 4

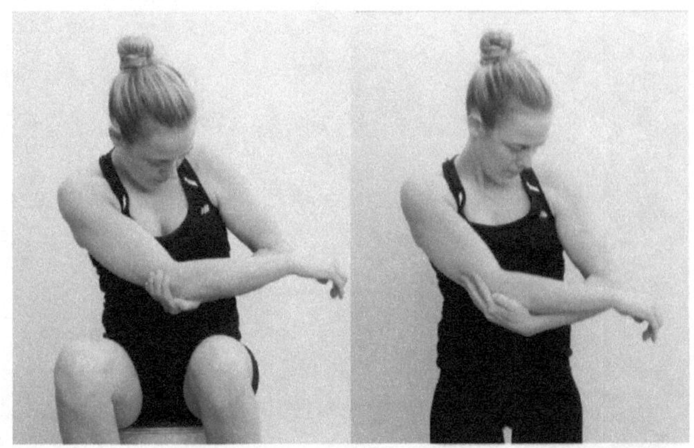

Exercise 5 Sitting   Exercise 5 Standing

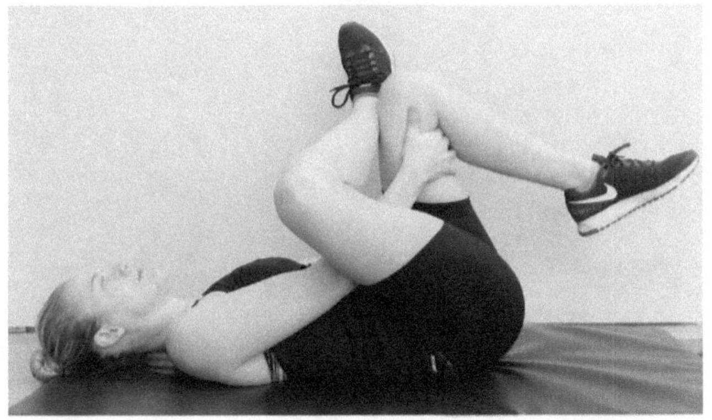

Exercise 6A

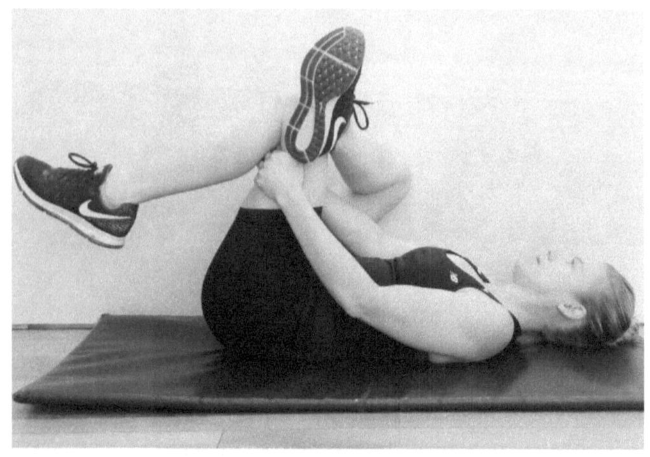

Exercise 6B

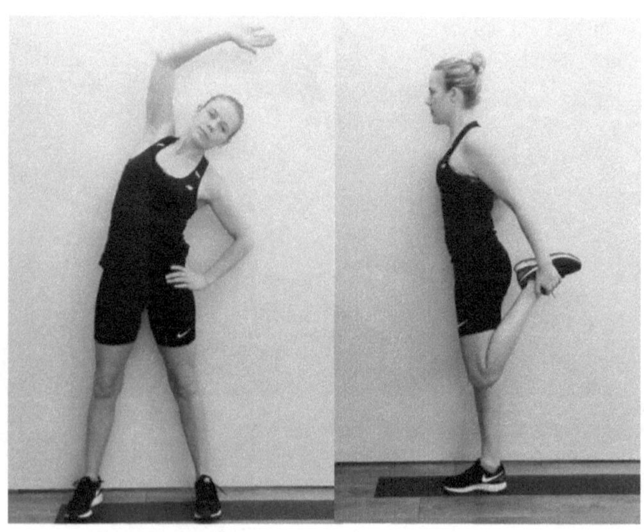

Exercise 7   Exercise 8

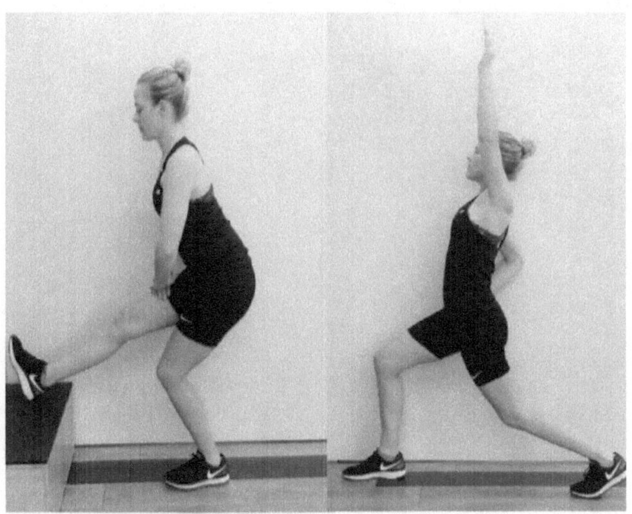

Exercise 9

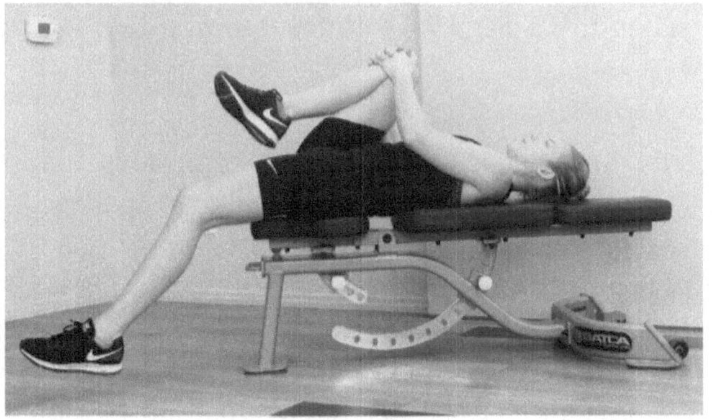

Exercise 10

173

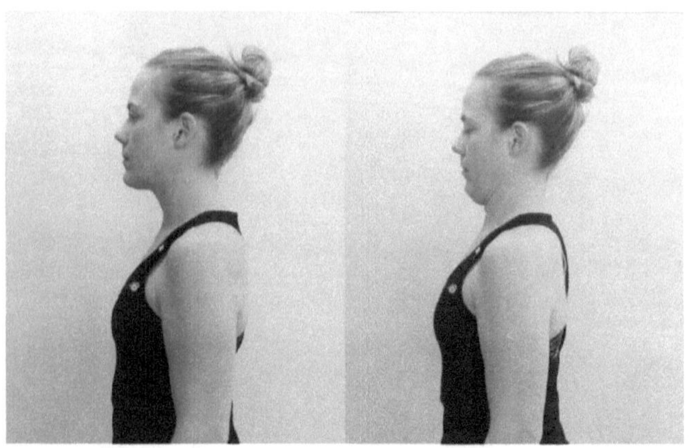

Exercise Chin Tuck A   Exercise Chin Tuck B

Chin tuck: This is a strengthening exercise more than a stretch. Tuck your chin directly inward and hold for 1 second. Repeat 10-15 times. Do <u>not</u> tuck your chin up or down.

There are various home care techniques that help increase flexibility and mobility. For instance, self-massage releases muscle tightness or trigger points and is an easy and effective technique. Trigger points are tender spots deep in the muscle representing adhesions or knots. Trigger points are typically caused by a sedentary lifestyle, poor nutrition, bad posture, stress, injuries and other lifestyle factors. Using a foam roller or pressure ball to assist in breaking up trigger points will help resume normal blood flow and function. When pressure is applied to a trigger point, pain can be experienced locally or referred to another area. The pain you experience while using a foam roller or pressure ball should be similar to the gentle pain you experience with stretching. It should be noticeable and slightly uncomfortable, but not intolerable. When you have completed your self-care you should feel better. Here are a few of our favorite foam roller and pressure ball positions. To see more, visit us online at familyhealthadvocacy.com.

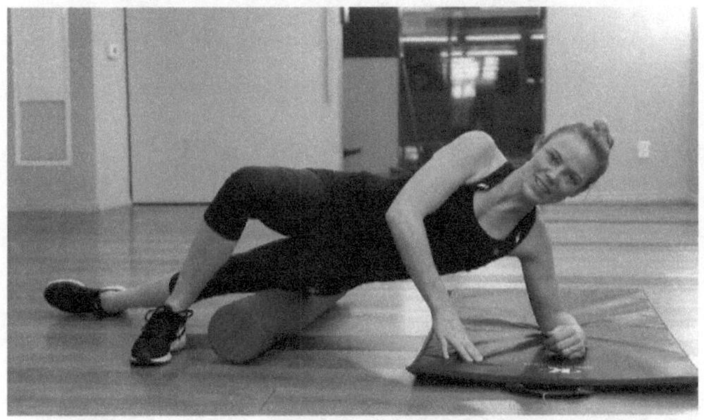

Foam Roll 1A

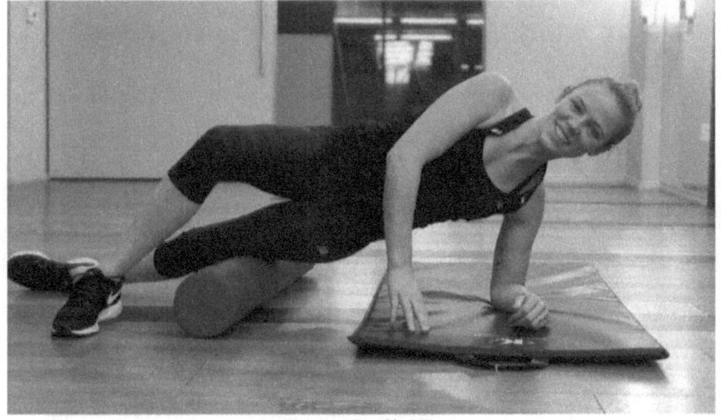

Foam Roll 1B

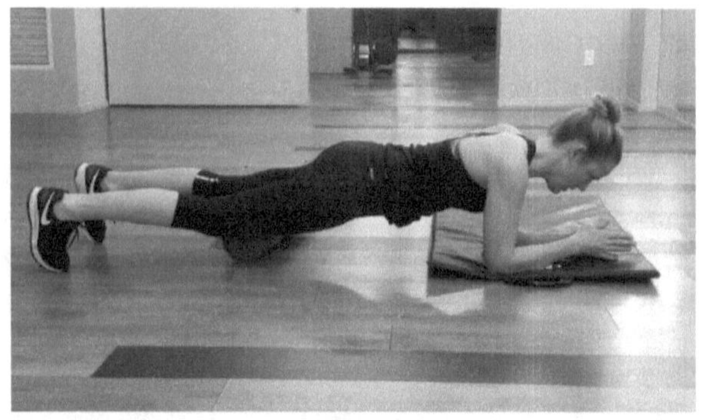

Foam Roll 2A

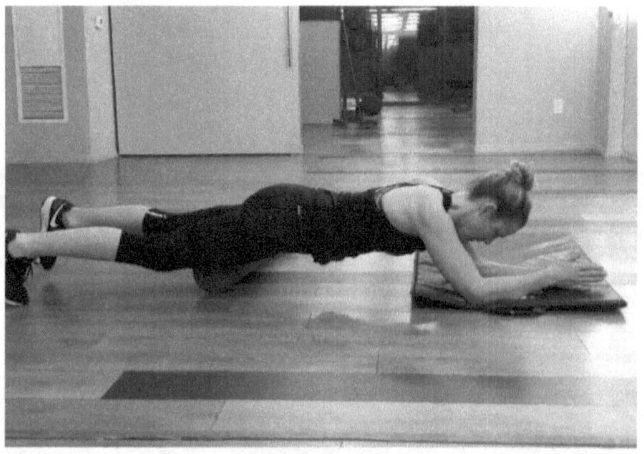

Foam Roll 2B

Position yourself on top of the foam roller and use the weight of your body to slowly roll back and forth over it, like a rolling pin. Try to allow your body to relax as much as possible over the roller. The above positions help to loosen muscles in your outer thigh, the iliotibial band and quadriceps. Roll each position for 3-5 minutes 1-2 times per day.

General Tips

- **Slow start:** Slow and steady wins the race! Doing too much too soon may result in more pain or injury. Doing something is better than nothing. If all you can manage is a five-minute walk, then take that five-minute walk. It's a start!
- **Move every day:** A little movement every day goes a long way. You don't need to do a full exercise routine each day, but you should stretch daily.
- **Be patient:** Fibromyalgia did not develop overnight, and healing won't be instantaneous either. It takes time. Be patient with your body.
- **Include your family and friends:** Recruiting accountability or workout partners helps you stay motivated and adds a social component to exercise!

"There is no magic drug against fibromyalgia, and in my opinion, there will never be...
aerobic exercise is the most effective weapon we have."

—Dr. Winfried Hauser, M.D

Bisma's Story

I'm a 23-year-old student. I used to experience chronic pain all over and get really bad headaches. I couldn't move very well and experienced stiffness everywhere.

Since following the program, my pain has reduced drastically, and the headaches are gone. The best part is that I am sleeping so much better. I had an amazing connection with Dr. Casey and Dr. Morgan. They have me doing all of the right exercises to help me and have taught me that I am able to solve the underlying problem, as well as heal through natural methods rather than medication. I recommend this program because there is so much for everyone to gain.

HEALTHCARE PRACTITIONERS

Getting Back to Our Roots

Humans have had a natural health philosophy and approach since the beginning of time. Communities such as the Okinawans, Hunzas, Vilcabambas, and Masai still often live to 100 years of age or more. They are truly living, and not merely surviving.

What we now call "alternative medicine" was mainstream until the invention of conventional medicine, when the use of drugs and surgery quickly replaced a self-healing approach to health. Today, there is a growing movement taking us back to our roots. Here are some additional natural healthcare options that will honour your body's self-healing ability.

Massage Therapy

Massage therapy can be beneficial for both acute and chronic conditions. Therapists can be helpful in the treatment of certain injuries and disabilities. Massage therapists are knowledgeable in physiology and anatomy and use specific techniques to treat their clients. Research supports the benefits of massage therapy for various conditions including pain, anxiety, and depression in fibromyalgia patients.

Acupuncture

Acupuncture is the insertion of thin metal needles to stimulate specific acupuncture points in the body. This regulates the energy flow of qi throughout the body and restores health to the mind and body. The needles are manipulated either by hand or by electrical stimulation, called electroacupuncture. While there is conflicting evidence of the benefits of acupuncture for treating fibromyalgia, there are countless reports from individuals who have benefited from acupuncture. Acupuncture is relatively painless and, when performed by a trained practitioner, has few risks.

Physiotherapy/Physical Therapy

Physiotherapy or physical therapy is treatment focused on restoring and maintaining the patient's mobility, function, and well-being. Patients are guided through physical rehabilitation, injury prevention, and experience increased health and fitness. This form of therapy has been shown to remove muscle stress, strengthen the body, and reduce fatigue in fibromyalgia patients.

Reflexology

Reflexology is when a practitioner applies focused pressure to specific points on the hands and feet. It works to affect tissues, glands, and organs by stimulating the electrical energy of the nervous system. The goal is to return the body to a state of homeostasis. Evidence supports reflexology as a great option to reduce fibromyalgia symptoms such as pain in multiple areas of the body.

Chiropractic

Chiropractic is an evidence-based, non-invasive, hands-on health care discipline that provides diagnosis and care of the neuromusculoskeletal system. Chiropractors focus on the diagnosis of misalignments of the joints, especially those of the spinal column, which may cause other disorders by affecting the nerves, muscles, and organs.

Osteopathy

Osteopathy is a hands-on therapy that focuses on somatic dysfunction or lack of balance in the joints, spine, muscles, vascular and lymphatic system. Osteopaths focus on slow and gentle manual readjustments to gently free restrictions to help restore balance in the body. Osteopaths tend to use only their hands, rather than tools.

Prolotherapy

Prolotherapy is a non-surgical therapy used to help strengthen or tighten weak or unstable ligaments or tendons. A stretched or torn ligament or tendon can result in chronic pain. Prolotherapy is the injection of a natural solution like glucose to trick the body into repairing itself. Prolotherapy works by stimulating the body's natural healing response which results in building new tissue in a weakened area. Temporary pain, stiffness, and swelling are often noted at the injection site. Prolotherapists may be trained osteopaths, medical doctors, or orthopedic physicians.

Functional Medicine

Functional medicine focuses on identifying and addressing the root cause of disease and proposing personalized treatments and lifestyle modifications. This therapy choice is gaining traction in the fibromyalgia community due to the success of treatment.

Naturopathic Medicine

Naturopathic medicine is a primary health care system that blends modern scientific knowledge with traditional and natural forms of medicine. Often naturopaths recommend specific diet and lifestyle changes to the patient, along with therapies including hydrotherapy, homeopathy, botanical medicine, traditional Chinese acupuncture, and more.

Biofeedback / Neurofeedback

During a biofeedback session, electrodes are attached to your skin or finger. The electrodes or sensors send signals to a monitor that indicates a stress response through changes such as body temperature, heart rate, and blood pressure. Several different relaxation exercises are used including deep breathing and progressive muscle relaxation. Biofeedback promotes relaxation and reduces stress.

Mindfulness

Mindfulness is the practice of being fully present. When we are present, we are aware of where we are and what we're doing. The technique is used by many practitioners in a variety of ways and reduces stress and anxiety that is often a result of regret and guilt over the past or fear of the future. Research shows mindfulness reduces stress and improves sleep in patients with fibromyalgia.

Cindy's Story

I'm a 49-year-old mother of two. I had been experiencing widespread pain all over my body for years. I tried everything, saw many doctors, and nothing helped. I had come to accept that I would have to deal with the pain for the rest of my life. My friend told me about Dr. Morgan and Dr. Casey and the success she had with her health from working with them. I was very skeptical but decided to follow their recommendations as a last resort. I'm so glad I did. The doctors also prescribed a specific exercise program for my problem. The changes in my mobility and flexibility were beyond my expectations at my age. I am now able to bend and lift, go up and down the stairs without the excruciating strain and pain I used to get. What's even more exciting is that the numbness and tingling in my hands and feet has completely disappeared! I would recommend this program to anyone because it works!

DRUGS

The number one cause of disease in western society is stress. There are three types of stress—physical, chemical, and emotional. Experiencing some stress is healthy, but we were never meant to experience and withstand the chronic and sustained physical strains, toxic overload, and emotional pressures that we experience in society today.

Things are only getting worse, hence the uprising of "millennial" conditions like fibromyalgia, chronic fatigue syndrome, and myofascial pain syndrome. The sad truth is that very few people see a holistic healthcare practitioner as their first line of defense when dealing with a health problem. Statistically speaking, most people attend their family physician first.

None of our patients with fibromyalgia have ever told us that their medical doctor gave them exercise or nutritional advice, discussed eliminating toxins, or suggested nurturing mindfulness. When seeing a medical doctor about a problem, their solution is always drugs.

Doctors often say they don't know what is causing fibromyalgia pain and that patients will simply have to learn to live with it or take medications to mask the symptoms. These medications often have side effects that include increased sensitization of pain, fatigue, or alteration of normal gut flora affecting digestive function. If the pre-existing symptoms are not masked by the medication, the mountain of symptoms grows, and it appears that the medication is making things worse. If the medication masks the symptoms and there are minimal or no side effects, it appears the problem is getting better. But what happens if you discontinue the medication? The symptoms return.

We get it! We know that there are times when prescription drugs are necessary and can be lifesaving. But in North America, we consume seventy-five percent of the world's prescription drugs. We have grown accustomed to taking medication as a first response to any symptom. Our healthcare system has turned into a sick care system. We don't give ourselves the time needed to honor our natural ability to heal.

Poor Health Isn't Due to a Lack of Drugs

A 2013 study by researchers with The Mayo Clinic found that seven out of ten Americans are on at least one prescription drug. That doesn't even include over-the-counter medications! In 2014, Express Scripts found the average American spends $1,370.00 each year on prescription medication. These stats are staggering and it's not getting better. *Consumer Reports* states that the number of prescriptions filled by American adults and children rose eighty-five percent between 1997 and 2016. It's no surprise that in 2014, nearly 1.3 million people sought emergency room treatment for adverse drug effects to properly prescribed medications and according to U.S. government data, 124,000 people died.

The quick fix of drugs is turning into a rapid downward spiral. People relying on medication often resort to taking more medication to mask the new side effect symptoms from the first drug, and many have to increase the strength or dosage because their body quickly becomes accustomed to the drugs.

You may start to feel better on medication but ask yourself what the toxins are doing to your body. Drugs may provide short-term benefits, but they also come with profound health risks. Consider all the other ways you can treat your symptoms that don't involve potentially dangerous pharmaceuticals.

Remember, all dis-ease comes from stress, including poor nutrition, chemical, emotional and physical stress. The true solution to an underlying problem is not always easy to find, especially with fibromyalgia. If your medical doctor won't help you find the cause, rather than merely masking the symptoms, we hope this book empowers you to take charge of your own healing journey and find solutions that help you get to the root of your symptoms.

We understand needing relief from your symptoms, but fibromyalgia is not a short-term problem, so why look for a short-term solution? The three main medications commonly prescribed to treat fibromyalgia do not solve the root cause; they simply try to trick your brain into not feeling the symptoms. Like anything else in life, turning a blind eye to the problem will only make things worse. If you don't fix that rattling sound under the hood of your car, do you think that problem will get better or worse? Your health is no different.

Few of these drugs have been carefully studied to see how they interact with one another, and unfortunately, more drugs mean more side effects and more health problems. To pharmaceutical companies, this just means more profit.

If you ever doubted that pharmaceutical companies are profit-driven rather than health-driven, consider that they spend significantly more money on marketing their drugs than they do on research and development to ensure they are safe and effective for consumption. Every single drug that has been pulled from the shelf because it is too dangerous was at one time passed by the FDA as being safe and effective.

Ask questions! Ask yourself, is this remedy addressing the underlying cause? There are no shortcuts to health. Make educated decisions. *You* are your own doctor!

There are two important factors to consider when evaluating the cost-benefit these drugs have on your health: Number Needed To Treat (NNT), and Number Needed To Harm (NNH).

NNT is the average number of people who need to be treated with the medication in order for one person to receive benefit. For example, if ten people need to be treated before one person receives a benefit, the NNT is ten. The lower the NNT number, the better.

NNH, on the other hand, is the number needed to harm. This is the measure of how many people need to be treated with the medication in order for one person to have an adverse reaction. For example, if seven people are treated in order for one person to experience an adverse reaction, the NNH is seven. The higher the NNH number, the better.

The Three Commonly Used Drugs for Fibromyalgia

Cymbalta

Cymbalta is a brand name of duloxetine, which is an antidepressant. Although researchers are not exactly certain how Cymbalta helps patients with fibromyalgia, they think that it may help calm down pain signals by increasing the level of serotonin and norepinephrine blocking it from re-entering cells.

The FDA approved Cymbalta in 2004 and when you visit their page you will find a highlighted warning at the top of the page reporting increased risk of suicidal thoughts and behavior: "WARNING: Suicidality and Antidepressant Drugs."

Cymbalta NNT: 8
Cymbalta NNH: 6-18

With the NNT of eight, for one person to achieve fifty percent reduction in pain, eight people would need to be treated. This means it takes eight people taking this drug in order for one person to benefit.

Lyrica

Lyrica is the brand-name of a drug that targets nerve signals. It is often used to relieve nerve pain for those with shingles and diabetic neuropathy and also used to treat partial seizures.

Scientists aren't exactly sure how Lyrica improves fibromyalgia symptoms, but it seems Lyrica helps decrease the number of nerve signals, calming down overly sensitive nerve cells.

Lyrica NNT: 10
Lyrica NNH: 11

In *Cochrane Clinicians*, Dr. Arnold, M.D., noted that the number needed to treat for pregabalin (the generic drug name of Lyrica) is 9.7 people in order to reduce pain for one person by fifty percent. Typically, Lyrica has to be taken in two pills a day for twelve weeks to see a benefit in one person. 168 pills per person multiplied by ten people is 1,680 pills needed to be taken by ten people to have one person benefit by fifty percent. Seems like there is one party benefiting the most—the pharmaceutical company!

Lyrica's number needed to harm is eleven, which means eleven people take the medication before someone is harmed. It's not surprising that most people discontinue using pregabalin because of adverse effects.

Savella

Savella is a selective serotonin and norepinephrine reuptake inhibitor. It is similar to drugs used to treat depression and other psychiatric disorders. The theory is that Savella increases the levels of neurotransmitters which may ease pain and reduce fatigue.

Savella NNT: 8-10

Savella NNH: 6

In order for someone to benefit from Savella, the number of patients needed to be treated ranges from eight to ten. The number of people treated before one person is harmed is six. If you parse this data, it means more users will be harmed than helped by this drug.

COMMON SYMPTOMS

A diagnosis of fibromyalgia usually comes as a result of a variety of common symptoms presenting themselves at once. Sometimes these symptoms are actually isolated, and by identifying each individual symptom a fibromyalgia patient can more easily regain their global sense of health.

Brain Fog

Brain fog is a common symptom in fibromyalgia patients and it's increasingly common among the under forty population. Brain fog affects memory, focus, and learning, as well as other cognitive dysfunctions, and it's not something that can be medically tested.

Brain fog symptoms include:

- Confusion
- Anxiety
- Trouble sleeping
- Irritability
- Low energy
- Fatigue
- Forgetfulness
- Low motivation

Causes of brain fog include:

- Stress
- Lack of physical exercise
- Inflammation
- Menopause
- Allergies
- Lack of sleep
- Poor diet and nutrition
- Dehydration
- Gluten sensitivity

If you are experiencing brain fog, stay positive! Many people have resolved it by applying the natural solutions we have discussed in this book – like sleep, nutrition, and exercise – which have been proven to improve memory, focus, and concentration.

Restless Leg Syndrome

Restless Leg Syndrome (RLS) is a condition that affects as many as 10% of adults. Many are even unaware that they have the condition. RLS, also referred to as Willis-Ekbom disease, is a nervous system condition that causes an irresistible urge to move your legs and a twitching of the muscles in the legs. RLS symptoms are characterized by an unpleasant feeling in the legs, and some even describe it as a crawling and creeping sensation on the feet and thighs.

While RLS symptoms can be felt throughout the day, most people experience symptoms at night when lying in bed. Because of this, it can cause difficulty sleeping and is now considered a sleep disorder. The condition affects two percent of children but the majority of those with RLS are adults. Many people who suffer from fibromyalgia also experience RLS.
RLS can have various causes, such as stress, lack of exercise, underlying medical conditions, iron deficiency, excessive smoking and alcohol consumption.

If you are experiencing any of the symptoms of RLS, visit your healthcare practitioner. Tests and a thorough medical history can help uncover the underlying problem. Various treatment methods are available and vary according to the cause and extent of the condition. Natural solutions that may help relieve symptoms of RLS include: cutting down on caffeine, tobacco and alcohol consumption; creating a healthy and regular bedtime ritual, as discussed in earlier sections; regular exercise; cold and hot compresses on the legs; meditation and deep breathing; taking magnesium, iron, and calcium supplements; and avoid medications.

Chronic Fatigue Syndrome

Chronic fatigue syndrome (CFS) is a complex chronic disorder characterized by extreme fatigue that isn't relieved by rest. The cause is not related to any underlying medical condition. People with CFS are frequently unable to perform their daily activities, and in some of the worst cases they can be confined to their beds. The condition affects millions of people all over the world, and women appear to be affected the most. CFS is a common symptom experienced by people with fibromyalgia.

There is no known cure for CFS, primarily because the underlying cause is so specific to the individual. Symptoms can last anywhere from months to years, but many people have resolved their condition – or at least significantly reduced their symptoms – by employing a range of natural solutions.

CFS: Causes

The cause of CFS is unknown as it varies according to each individual, but research shows many contributing factors which include:

- Viral infections
- Weak immune system
- Hormonal imbalances
- Stress
- Depression and anxiety

CFS: Symptoms

The symptoms of CFS will vary in every individual and range in severity. The most prominent symptom is, of course, fatigue. A frustrating factor is that the fatigue doesn't get relieved by rest. Other symptoms include sleep disorders, pain, cognitive impairment, anxiety, depression, flu-like symptoms, body temperature changes, and stress.

CFS: Diagnosis

Diagnosing CFS can take time because the symptoms can mimic other medical conditions, so doctors must rule out all other illnesses in order to diagnose CFS. Be sure to see your healthcare practitioner if you have experienced chronic fatigue or any of the above symptoms for more than six months. A review of your full health history including any medications you may be taking should also be discussed. It's important to be thorough, as any missing information may hinder your ability to uncover the underlying cause of your condition.

Natural Solutions for CFS

There is no specific cure for CFS, but there are various natural solutions that patients use to help alleviate their symptoms. In some cases, these therapies even resolve the condition. It is always a good idea to discuss your natural approach with your healthcare provider.

Physical Activity

The best natural remedy for CFS is exercise. It's especially important to engage in aerobic activity in order to raise your heart rate. Exercises such as swimming, walking, and climbing stairs should not add to the fatigue you already have. Always start with just a few minutes of exercise and gradually increase.

Cognitive Behavioral Therapy

This therapy focuses on helping a patient accept the condition, manage the symptoms, and change their attitude towards the condition. Cognitive Behavioral Therapy is offered on a one to one basis, just like seeing a psychotherapist, so it is important to work with a trained and experienced practitioner.

Lifestyle Changes

By this, we mean changing your routines and schedule in order to incorporate rest and relaxation into your day. Eliminating stressors can have a huge impact in reducing fatigue. However, make sure that you do not sleep too much during the day.

Decrease the Consumption of Caffeine & Alcohol

If you have CFS, you should eliminate caffeine and alcohol as they can aggravate your symptoms and interfere with the natural balance of the body.

Leaky Gut

Recent studies identify a connection between chronic pain conditions like fibromyalgia and a leaky gut, which is an intestinal permeability disorder. This condition is a recent phenomenon, and ongoing research is being conducted to help health practitioners fully understand it and better assist their patients.

Intestinal lining is meant to act as a barrier to prevent toxins and bacteria from travelling from the gut into the bloodstream. However, sometimes the gut may develop small fissures, allowing food, toxins, and other elements to penetrate into the blood. This can lead to inflammations, which can result in digestive problems as well as other chronic conditions, including fibromyalgia.

Everyone has a certain degree of a leaky gut since the intestinal lining is not completely impermeable. However, some people may experience changes which may alter their digestive system resulting in the cracks or holes in the gut lining. Other common causes of a leaky gut include:

- Heavy alcohol consumption
- Chronic stress
- Medications
- Poor nutrition

Chronic pain, fibromyalgia, arthritis, asthma, acne, and obesity are among the significant conditions linked to leaky gut syndrome. Healthcare practitioners are now focusing on ways in which they can heal the gut in order to resolve these symptoms, and proper nutrition is one important method. Eliminating processed and inflammatory foods, medications, alcohol, and addressing food allergies are key. Regular exercise and stress have proven to help treat this condition and rebuild the gut to its original state.

Carpal Tunnel Syndrome

Carpal Tunnel Syndrome is an incredibly frustrating condition that frequently disrupts a person's ability to get quality sleep, perform their job, and do simple daily activities. Carpal Tunnel Syndrome is common in fibromyalgia sufferers. It's a condition that is most frequently characterized by pain in the wrist, where the carpal tunnel is located, but can also include symptoms of pins and needles or numbness in the hands, fingers, and arms. In advanced cases some people have difficulty grasping objects or even holding a glass of water.

The Source of Carpal Tunnel

The wrist and elbow are potential nerve entrapment sites causing symptoms of Carpal Tunnel and need to be examined by a qualified healthcare practitioner. However, a commonly overlooked source of carpal tunnel symptoms come from nerve roots in the neck. In fact, a study in The Lancet journal showed that up to 75% of carpal tunnel patients had a nerve problem in their neck. Anyone displaying these symptoms should have their spine and nervous system assessed by a chiropractor.

Unfortunately, many people are immediately prescribed medication or even surgery to deal with their symptoms. With the many Carpal Tunnel Syndrome cases reportedly being mis-diagnosed, these procedures offer little help and have the potential to make matters worse.

What does this have to do with fibromyalgia? Well, studies have shown that there is a high prevalence of Carpal Tunnel Syndrome in patients with fibromyalgia. Both conditions are common in middle-aged and older women. Among those women with Carpal Tunnel Syndrome, nearly 50% have fibromyalgia as well. Fibromyalgia is considered a significant risk factor for Carpal Tunnel Syndrome because of the increased pain sensitivity that accompanies fibromyalgia, increasing one's susceptibility to carpal tunnel from repetitive strain and poor posture.

What does food have to do with it?

There is a strong possibility that there is a nutritional component to Carpal Tunnel Syndrome. In fact, the symptoms could be due to nutritional deficiencies or heavy metal toxicity. Studies have linked deficiencies of vitamin B, D, magnesium, and zinc to Carpal Tunnel Syndrome and fibromyalgia.

If all of this fails, it's time to consider having your levels tested for heavy metal toxins. This can be resolved with a heavy metal detox program, so revisit that chapter in this book if this speaks to you.

Get to the root of it!

The important thing is to get to the root cause of the problem. If you do, you should be able to get your life back in a matter of weeks and enjoy all that life has to offer. Whatever you do, don't neglect the problem. Take action now!

CONCLUSION

Congratulations! Making it this far shows your true commitment to your health. By now you may have already started making changes to your lifestyle and creating healthy habits. You may already be experiencing the benefits of those choices. If you haven't started to take action, stop waiting, the time is now! Go back and read chapter three, "A Healthy Mind," and read it as many times as it takes in order for you to take action.

We hope you enjoyed reading this book and found the content to be interesting, but more importantly we hope it's given you practical ideas and solutions to take control of your journey to health. We wrote this book to give you tangible and practical action steps for you to put to work. With the information covered in this book, as well as our online course and community, you have all you need to free yourself from the shackles of fibromyalgia and enjoy a life of health.

Our hope is that you will join our mission and share this book and its information with other fibromyalgia sufferers and anyone else that may benefit. Health information is always changing, and we strive to always be there as a resource for you, your family, and friends.

Your health is your most valuable asset and the time you invest in it is worth every second. If nothing else, this will allow you to enjoy each day more and raise your quality of life as you begin to do the things you love again.

Consider this book your health manual moving forward. Treat it as your reference book to assure you remain on track. To remain up to date with cutting-edge health information, please join us in our online community. There you will be able to discuss any health challenges you may have and also celebrate your successes with us and other people just like you.